HEALTH CARE MANAGEMENT
IN
PHYSICAL THERAPY

HEALTH CARE MANAGEMENT IN PHYSICAL THERAPY

By

MARK A. BRIMER, P.T., M.B.A.

Illustrations by
John F. Braun

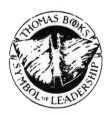

CHARLES C THOMAS • PUBLISHER
Springfield • Illinois • U.S.A.

Published and Distributed Throughout the World by

CHARLES C THOMAS • PUBLISHER
2600 South First Street
Springfield, Illinois 62794-9265

© *1990 by* CHARLES C THOMAS • PUBLISHER

ISBN 0-398-05642-0

Library of Congress Catalog Card Number: 89-20347

With THOMAS BOOKS *careful attention is given to all details of manufacturing
and design. It is the Publisher's desire to present books that are satisfactory as to their
physical qualities and artistic possibilities and appropriate for their particular use.*
THOMAS BOOKS *will be true to those laws of quality that assure a good name
and good will.*

Printed in the United States of America
SC-R-3

Library of Congress Cataloging-in-Publication Data

Brimer, Mark A.
  Health care management in physical therapy / by Mark A. Brimer ;
illustrations by John F. Braun.
      p.   cm.
  Includes bibliographical references.
  ISBN 0-398-05642-0
  1. Physical therapy services—Administration.   I. Title.
  [DNLM: 1. Health Sciences—organization and administration.
2. Physical Therapy.   WB 460 B857h]
RM701.B74   1990
362.1'78—dc20
DNLM/DLC
for Library of Congress   89-20347
                                                                        CIP

To my wife Leslee,
my parents,
and sons Eric and Christopher

INTRODUCTION

The focus of this book is on physical therapists as supervisors in all health care settings. This includes hospitals, nursing homes, home health agencies, rehabilitation centers, and in the private practice setting. Many physical therapists have been placed in these supervisory positions as a result of outstanding job performance and a willingness to guide other health care professionals in providing quality patient care.

In most instances, however, the professional has little educational background concerning the proper methods to use in health care management. As a result, the new or inexperienced supervisor is often confronted with the need to be an effective manager while at the same time trying to understand the complex human relationships that are frequently encountered within the working environment. The supervisor soon recognizes that his or her former position of employment, as a staff physical therapist, has changed from one of solely providing patient care to one of becoming a leader of a group of health care professionals. Thus, the primary goal changes from one of an individual working with patients to an individual attempting to get things done with and through other people.

For the physical therapist, health care management can be both difficult and personally rewarding. The purpose of this text is to guide the physical therapist through the ever-increasing demands of health care supervision. As such, the book is introductory, in that it assumes no previous knowledge of the proper methods to use in managing health care employees. The book will be of value to the physical therapist who has recently accepted a managerial position and is concerned about the potential problems to be encountered and how they might best be solved. For the experienced supervisor, the book is intended to refresh their thinking and provide a new and challenging look at both their own position and that of their employees in providing quality patient care.

It is important to recognize that the position as supervisor is one of the most critical roles a physical therapist can assume. Accepting and properly performing the managerial function of supervision means the daily responsibility of guiding a department or practice towards desired objectives and goals. In large institutions, such as a hospital, the supervisor must contend not only with the fellow employees but also with patients and relatives under conditions which may make supervision very difficult. The supervisor is often torn between satisfying the role as a health care professional and satisfying the requirements of being a supervisor. The demands made by the administration of the institution, as well as by medical doctors, can pull the supervisor in any number of directions further complicating that role.

The changing health care environment is also having an impact on the management of the health care employee. Providing health care services is becoming increasingly more complex as a result of government regulations concerning the provision of health care and the rapid advances of medical science and technology. Today, the physical therapist must not only continue to provide high-quality rehabilitative services but also keep abreast of the latest diagnostic techniques and procedures available for patient treatment. The supervisor also has the added responsibility of attempting to satisfy the demands of those organizations, such as insurance companies, who are responsible for absorbing the cost of rehabilitative services provided to the patient.

Coordinating these processes is a demanding requirement for the supervisor. This book provides material which is based upon the research of a number of experts in the fields of management, behavorial science, and the social sciences. The modern health care supervisor must have considerable knowledge of the human aspects of supervision and the behavorial and social factors that help motivate employees. Although the book does not cover every aspect of health care management, it does provide a balanced picture of the role the physical therapy supervisor plays in providing quality patient care while continuing to meet the objectives and goals of the health care organization.

CONTENTS

ix

HEALTH CARE MANAGEMENT
IN
PHYSICAL THERAPY

Chapter One

HEALTH CARE MANAGEMENT

THE PRACTICE OF MANAGEMENT

Many physical therapists have either consciously or unconsciously planned a career in health care management. Upon graduation from professional training, the physical therapist typically accepts a position within a health care organization that is non-managerial in nature. As the physical therapist becomes established in a career, often the first promotion will be to a position where the job responsibility includes supervising other health care professionals.

Once promoted to a supervisory position, the physical therapist, as a health care professional, has embarked on a management career. It is from this point on that the physical therapist will be accomplishing the objectives of the health care organization through other health care professionals.

Health care managers and organizations go together hand in hand. The need for managers arises because health care organizations exist. While the health care organizations' managers are not the only vital resource, they do have a significant impact on the organizations' success and the quality of health care provided.

Since managers have a significant influence on organizational success, good ones are continually in demand. As a result of high demand, top health care managers are often paid very well. The manager of the Humana Corporation, one of the largest for-profit hospital chains in America, received a 1987 salary and bonus totaling $867,000.[1] Hospital administrators of medium-sized hospitals frequently receive salaries of $80,000 or more. Of course, managers of small health care organizations and those at levels below top administration will earn considerably less.

Well beyond the year 2000, the demand for health care will continue to rise. As the population of elderly individuals continues to grow, along with further increases in life expectancy, there will be a greater demand for health care services and managers to organize its delivery. By the year 2020, it has been projected that 44.3 percent of the population of the United States will be between the ages of 65 and 84.[2]

This book is about how health care organizations are managed and how the physical therapist can take an active role in setting and achieving goals within the organization. The health care supervisor gives direction to other professionals and non-professionals that they manage. They must think through the organization's goals and determine the resources essential to achieve results. The health care manager must lead employees toward productivity and be responsible for the social impact their organization has on society. Helping you understand how the health care manager accomplishes these different tasks is the purpose of this book. It is not the intent of this book to include every potential problem a health care manager may face but, rather, to provide all health care managers with insight into modern health care management principles, regardless of the individual's background, training, goals, or the size of the health care organization.

WHAT IS HEALTH CARE MANAGEMENT?

Health care management is the process of coordinating human and non-human resources to accomplish the objectives and goals of the organization. Health care managers will achieve institutional objectives and goals by arranging for others to perform organizational activities.

Management is essential to providing the coordination of effort towards producing quality patient care. Managers perform many complex and interrelated activities. Some of the most common activities performed by all health care managers include:

- Setting the objectives of the organization.
- The formulation of plans to achieve organizational objectives.
- Identifying the activities which are to be performed.
- Organizing individuals into groups.
- Defining the health care tasks to be performed.
- Determining the appropriate compensation levels for jobs.
- Acquiring health care personnel.
- Providing incentives to stimulate quality patient care.
- Measuring the achievement of objectives.
- Taking appropriate action if objectives are not achieved according to pre-established standards

Health care managers work with and through other health care professionals. They are often expected to accomplish more than other members of the organization. Good health care managers have the technical, professional and clinical competence to direct a department and the health care organization properly.

Thus, the job of a health care manager is a demanding one. The health care manager is usually evaluated on how well tasks are accomplished and how well the department or practice achieves designated objectives and goals. Above all, the health care manager is responsible for the actions of his or her subordinates. A health care manager's success or failure is dependent upon not only his or her own work but also the work of others within the organization.

MANAGERS IN HEALTH CARE ORGANIZATIONS

The term *health care management* has been defined as anyone who is responsible for supervising subordinates and the resources of the organization. In any health care organization there are varying types of managers with diverse responsibilities. Throughout this book, the terms *manager* and *supervisor* will be used interchangeably. The terms, as such, are to be recognized as synonymous.

Health care managers in all organizations are classified by their level in the organization and by the range of activities they perform and are ultimately responsible for. The common classifications to be used are: top management, middle level management, and first level management. The distinction between these classifications is demonstrated in Figure 1-1.

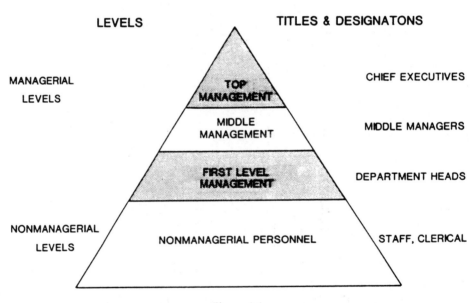

Figure 1-1.

Top Managers

In virtually all health care organizations, top management is responsible for the direction and overall management of the organization.

Typical titles of hospital personnel in top management positions include chief executive officer, president, or vice-president. Those individuals who occupy top management positions serve to interact with government agencies and represent the organization in community affairs. Major decisions involving the acquisition of new hospital equipment or the expansion of the present facility are also within the scope of their decision-making authority. It is not uncommon for top managers to spend most of their working day with peers and others outside the organization. Outside contacts can include meetings with community leaders, attorneys, and members of the medical community. They tend to spend little time with subordinates, unless it involves presenting awards for special recognition or attending hospital social functions. Almost all long-range planning and strategic decision making is handled by those in top management positions.

Middle Level Management

Physical therapists who are located in positions of middle management direct the activities of other managers. The title "Director of Rehabilitative Services" often reflects the distinction of a middle manager. In health care, the primary function of a middle manager would be to act as a buffer between first level management and the members of top management. As such, the middle manager directs activities which serve to implement organizational policies. The director of rehabilitative services may oversee the departments of physical therapy, occupational therapy, speech therapy, and the other rehabilitative services offered within the organization. The middle level manager's primary function would be to assist the directors of the other departments, guiding them in their decision making, and evaluating their overall performance.

First Level Management

The primary level of supervision in a health care organization is where the individual is responsible for managing the quality of health care services provided to the patient. The health care manager who is a first level manager is responsible for the direction of department employees. The individual at this level has no responsibility for supervising other health care managers except, possibly, an assistant director. In the hospital or rehabilitation center setting, a physical therapist as a first level manager would often be entitled "Director of Physical Therapy" or "Chief Physical Therapist." The manager supervises the activities of employees and participates in setting the direction and goals of the health care services to be provided.

MANAGERIAL LEVELS AND SKILL REQUIREMENTS

At each level of management a different set of skills is required to deal effectively with the numerous challenges presented in providing health care services. Robert Katz has identified three basic skills needed to be successful in management.[3] The three skills needed by all managers, regardless of their position in the organization are: technical, human, and conceptual skill. The amount of each of these skills needed by a manager will depend upon the managerial level (top, middle or lower level management), his or her responsibilities, and the role of the manager. At the lower levels of health care management, the supervisor will require more technical skill than any other type. Those individuals in middle management require more human relations skill. The importance of conceptual skill is primarily evidenced at top management positions. The distinction between these classifications is demonstrated in Figure 1-2.

SKILLS NEEDED FOR SUCCESSFUL MANAGEMENT

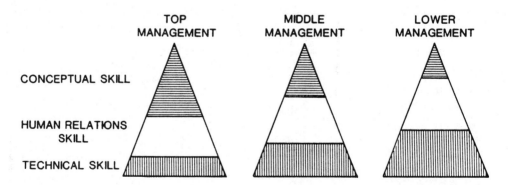

Figure 1-2.

Technical Skill

Technical skill is the ability to perform specialized activities in a given field. An orthopaedic surgeon, for example, requires a high degree of technical skill in order to properly and safely perform a total knee replacement. A physical therapist receives a high degree of specialized training in rehabilitation. This training includes a thorough understanding of the proper procedures and techniques to be used for the most beneficial patient outcome.

For the physical therapist, as a first level manager, technical skill will be of great importance since the supervisor must have a thorough understanding of how to perform the various jobs within the department. Unless the physical therapist has well-developed technical skills, the individual will not understand how and why things operate as they do. This, in turn, will have a profound impact on the therapist's ability to instruct others in proper performance. First level managers require high technical skills to evaluate patient treatment methods and direct the level of care offered by the department or practice. If the physical therapist does not thoroughly understand what patient treatment services are being offered by the department, he or she cannot assist the new or untrained worker in proper patient care. The importance of the technical skill is evidenced when supervising a new employee who is unfamiliar with a method of patient treatment. The first level manager should be prepared to teach the principles as well as the proper application of any service offered to the patient.

Human Relations Skill

Human relations skill is the ability to motivate, lead, understand, and work with other people as individuals or as groups. Human relations skill is of vital importance to the health care manager, since it serves to build a cooperative effort within the health care team. In comparison to the manager's need to have technical ability to work with the operations and procedures of a profession, human relations skill is especially useful when working with people.

Health care managers with a highly developed human relations skill are aware of their own attitudes as well as their beliefs about other individuals. This increased awareness enables them to see how their individual perceptions, beliefs, and viewpoints differ from those of others.

Managers who are aware of their own beliefs and those of their subordinates are able to blend the two in a manner that creates trust and understanding among all members of the working group.

At each level of management, the health care manager must have human relations skill. As can be evidenced in Figure 1-3, the need for human relations skill changes little in each of the three levels of management. The need for technical skill decreases dramatically as one progresses from lower level management to top management. Conceptual skills are of utmost importance at the level of top management.

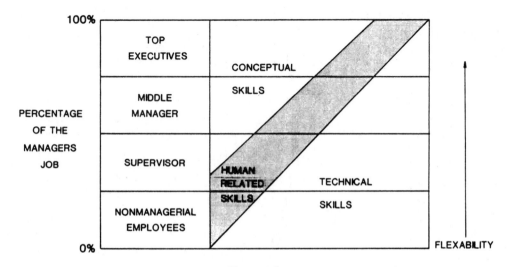

Figure 1-3.

Some physical therapists, in managerial positions, are able to develop human relations skill rapidly. These are individuals who easily understand the feelings of others and can develop an appreciation for events occurring within the organization. For those physical therapists who are lacking the basics in human relations skill, there are substantial gains to be derived from working with a department director who has mastered this ability. This informal on-the-job training can also be supplemented with course work at the graduate level. Many colleges offer programs in business administration. Courses in personnel management or human relations will often be of substantial benefit to the inexperienced manager.

When studying human relations skill, the physical therapist must recognize the two skills which are required. There are those skills which are required for managing problems that occur within a group. These are called intragroup skills. There are also intergroup skills which are required for handling problems which occur between groups. Intragroup skills are of prime importance to first level and middle management, whereas intergroup skills are important to top managers.

Conceptual Skill

Conceptual skills are those abilities that help the manager see the organization as a whole. Conceptual skill is mental, in that it involves the health care manager's ability to understand how an organization's various parts depend on each other and how a change in a given area can affect the organization as a whole.

A health care manager's conceptual skill becomes more important at the upper levels of the health care administration. The higher the manager is in the organization, the more the individual will be involved in planning and setting the direction of the organization. For the physical therapist aspiring to assume a top management position, conceptual skill will probably be the most important of all. Conceptual skill allows the individual the opportunity to assess potential changes in the health care environment. The ability to predict change and react in an appropriate fashion is part of the top manager's job.

THE COMPLEX ROLES OF THE HEALTH CARE SUPERVISOR

Through close examination of the job of almost any health care supervisor, it becomes readily apparent that it involves four major roles. The first role is that of being a good manager to all employees who work in the health care organization. The manager must have the professional and clinical competence to run the department in an organized fashion and see to it that the employees perform their assigned tasks.

The second role involves that of being a good subordinate to the supervisor to whom the individual manager must report. In an organization such as a hospital or rehabilitation center, the physical therapy supervisor will report to the top administrator or to one of the associate administrators. The physical therapist, as a supervisor, will be expected to be a good employee and follow the suggestions and recommendations of the supervisor or executive to whom he or she must ultimately report.

The third role provided by the supervisor of a physical therapy department is that of a connecting link between the administration of the organization and the employees who are members of the physical therapy department. In this position, the employees will recognize the department supervisor as part of the administration of the organization. For many employees, the department supervisor will be the only contact they have with any member of top management.

The fourth role the supervisor plays within the modern health care organization is that of a liaison between the supervisors of all other departments. The role here is to be supportive and actively work to coordinate services between the other departments. All departments should work together in an effort to continually improve the quality of health care provided to the patient and the community at large.

The intricate role of the health care supervisor can be further examined by referring to Figure 1-4. In this diagram, the role of the supervisor can be seen as a continual relationship with both horizontal and vertical dimensions. In the vertical direction, the supervisor must maintain good relations with the employees below and with the administration above. The supervisor must also engage in productive interactions with other departments in the organization. As a result of the complexity of relationships, the role as a department director or first line supervisor is often a difficult one. Here, the supervisor must not only accept responsibility for the actions of the members of the department but also must take at least partial responsibility for the functioning of the institution. The supervisor must continually strive to create good relations with the members of the medical staff, top management, fellow employees, patients, other department supervisors, and the local community.

Specifically, the individual who supervises the physical therapy department may perform a number of the following functions on any given day. For example, the supervisor has the daily responsibility of overseeing that the department complies with the treatment orders of physicians. This responsibility includes the proper scheduling of patients and the delivery of rehabilitative services. Additionally, the physical therapy supervisor may be requested to attend a meeting with other department supervisors sponsored by the administration of the hospital. Once the meeting has been concluded, the supervisor will determine whether or not the information should be relayed to subordinates at an informal meeting within the department.

The performance of these roles is not an activity which can be separated. In health care management, a role is defined as an organized set of observable behaviors that are attributed to a specific office or position.

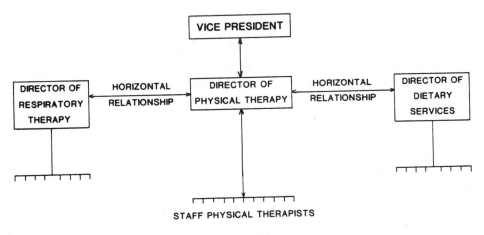

Figure 1-4.

As such, the manager may wear "a number of hats" in the performance of the job.

THE HEALTH CARE MANAGERIAL FUNCTIONS

Earlier in this chapter health care management was defined as the process of coordinating human and non-human resources to accomplish the objectives and goals of the organization. The process of coordinating resources requires that a manager perform a number of functions. One of the earliest classifications of the managerial functions was made by Henri Fayol, Europe's most distinguished contributor to the field of management theory and practice up to the middle of the present century. Fayol identified the five functions as planning, organizing, commanding, coordinating, and controlling.[4] Although the labeling of these functions has changed somewhat since Fayol's time, there is still a basic agreement about what the managerial functions are and how they can be performed.

Regardless of the type of health care organization, industry, or level of management hierarchy, there are at least five functions which must be performed by anyone who is a manager. They are: planning, organizing, staffing, controlling, and influencing. If an individual does not perform all of these functions to at least a certain extent, then he or she is not a manager in the true sense of the word. These functions are performed by all managers whenever and wherever there are organized groups of people.

Planning

Planning is the managerial function of deciding in advance what is to be done in the future. Planning is mental work, in that it is concerned with establishing the objectives to be achieved and allocating the proper resources to accomplish the established objectives. In health care, as well as in business or industry, planning must come before any of the other managerial functions. After the initial plans are established, the health care manager may proceed with the remaining managerial functions. Planning, as such, serves to determine the framework by which the other managerial functions are to be carried out. This is especially true for the physical therapist in a managerial position. Planning is a continuous process which, to be effective, must be performed on a daily basis. It is important to recognize that the planning function does not end when the manager begins to perform the four remaining functions. In the daily process of planning, the physical therapist must anticipate future problems, analyze them, assess their potential impact on employees and patients, and decide an appropriate course of action.

Managers at all levels in an organization actively participate in the planning process. Plans developed by those individuals in top management positions will be more in-depth and far-reaching than those developed at lower levels of the organization. Plans developed by top management will also be broader in scope than those made by others in the organization. The hospital's chief executive officer will devise plans for the entire organization, wheras the supervisor of the physical therapy department will prepare plans which enable the department to operate more efficiently and provide improved patient care.

Developing Short-Term and Long-Term Plans

In the health care environment, as well as in business and industry, there will be the development of two sets of plans for an organization, namely: short-term and long-term plans. Many factors influence who develops long- or short-term plans. The most common influencing factors are the supervisor's position in the health care organization and the type of health care services offered. Short-term plans are defined as those plans which cover a period of no longer than one year. Long-range plans extend beyond one year and may extend to five, ten, or even twenty years in advance (Figure 1-5).

Top managers, such as the chief executive officer or the chairman of

---

WHO PERFORMS LONG AND
SHORT RANGE PLANNING?

SHORT RANGE PLANS – Usually cover a period of time up to one year. Developed most often by Department Managers.

LONG RANGE PLANS – May cover a period of 5, 10 or even 20 years. Most often developed as part of the planning process of the top Administrators.

Figure 1-5.

the board, often develop plans which are fundamental and far reaching. Individuals in top management positions are concerned with the overall aspects of planning for the entire health care institution. As the supervisor of a physical therapy department, you will most likely be responsible for developing short-term plans of approximately one year. These plans may include projecting future staff requirements, changes in patient treatment patterns, or developing a departmental budget. There are also other activities such as planning the daily patient treatment schedule, setting employee work schedules or planning the schedule of preventative maintenance on the department's equipment which are considered short term in nature. The managerial development of short-term plans is vital to ensuring the various jobs within the department are done promptly, effectively, and on a daily basis.

Planning at all levels of health care management must be done with anticipation of future events. As is already well known, the future of health care is uncertain. The rapid changes in patient care in just the last ten years make it almost impossible for the supervisor to make anything other than broad assumptions about the future. In most health care settings it is strictly top management which assesses the future and develops long-range forecasts. Once forecasts have been developed by top management, individual supervisors take the responsibility for planning the implementation of change in their departments.

It is the supervisor's ultimate responsibility to develop plans which efficiently utilize the departmental space provided, the materials and supplies available, and provide for the best use of the employee's time. All management planning efforts should be concerned with the potential effects the plans may have on other members or departments within the organization. The success or failure of any plan will depend upon the reactions of those involved in its implementation. As supervisor of a physical therapy department, you must consider the potential impact of any plan on employees, directors or other departments, and even your own boss. The best plans have the total support of all individuals who will be involved in the final implementation process.

Developing Primary and Secondary Objectives

Part of the planning process of any health care organization is the development of primary and secondary objectives. Determining primary objectives is the responsibility of top management within the health care organization. Primary objectives outline the goals and end result toward which all plans and activities are to be directed. The objectives developed will constitute the purpose of the organization. For example, the overall top management objective for a hospital is to "care for the sick, help in the prevention of illness, provide quality care, and educate the community in health-related matters." A rehabilitation hospital might state as its primary objective to "provide total care to individuals with varying degrees of disability with a focus on providing services which enable them to achieve a maximum level of recovery or rehabilitation." Other primary objectives can include "practicing the best possible medicine," "operating without a loss," or "being a good place to work."

Secondary objectives are frequently developed by individual departments within the organization. Secondary objectives are important, since each department must have guidelines by which to operate. Secondary objectives are not as broad as primary objectives and therefore serve as specific guides for performance. Suppose, for example, one of the stated objectives of a hospital physical therapy department was "to provide patients with information regarding the profession of physical therapy." Obviously, this objective is much narrower than the one developed by top management in the hospital. It does, however, accomplish part of the primary goal of "educating the community in health-related matters." The contribution that secondary objectives make is the only means by which a primary objective can be accomplished (Figure 1-6).

It is essential for all supervisors to educate their employees as to the

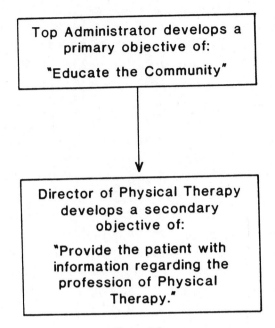

Figure 1-6.

differences between primary and secondary objectives. Employees should clearly understand not only the objectives of their own department but also those of the health care organization. Employees who fully understand how an assigned task fits into the scheme of the entire organization will be more committed to their respective jobs. In final analysis, the successful completion of any task ultimately depends upon a thorough understanding of its purpose by those individuals who are expected to carry it out. Once subordinates understand the organization's plans and objectives, they will be more committed to achieving specific organizational objectives and goals.

Organizing

Organizing involves the assignment of duties and activities that are required to achieve the health care organization's objectives and goals. Organizing plots the activities needed to accomplish objectives. It then combines the activities into work groups and assigns the responsibility for accomplishing them to subordinates. The managerial function of organizing provides the structure by which work can be coordinated and patient care can be delivered.

The chief executive officer is primarily the one who is charged with determining the structure for the organization. It is important, however, that each level of health care management understand how the organization has been structured, since it will provide the individual supervisor with a guide to organizing his or her own department. Every health care manager will be given the responsibility of determining the methods by which work is to be accomplished within the department. The top manager may establish the organization's formal structure, but it is the middle and first level managers who must make it functional.

To establish an organizational structure, the institution must first be departmentalized. The process of departmentalization arises from the division of work, which simply divides a job into more specialized component parts. Dividing work into smaller components results in greater efficiency, since each person is performing a smaller specialized part of the entire job. A group of people, each performing a specialized part of a job, can accomplish more than the same size group where each individual is trying to do the whole job alone. Suppose, for example, that a staff physical therapist, in addition to his or her own responsibilities, tried to perform all the functions performed by the occupational therapist, the social worker, and the nursing unit. In this case, little would get accomplished since the task would be so overwhelming. Therefore, dividing rehabilitation into component parts allows the attainment of far superior treatment results.

The process of dividing work into smaller activities allows the grouping together of similar functions. To create a department means to group individuals together who perform similar activities and to have them supervised by someone familiar with those activities. Health care institutions group individuals into major departments on the basis of function, product, territory, customer, process and equipment, or time.

By Function

Most departments within a hospital or a similar health care facility are grouped according to function. Grouping by function places all activities that are similar under one individual for direct supervision. Physical therapists are frequently grouped together in the department of physical therapy. Occupational therapists, social workers, speech therapists, as well as many others are also grouped in the same manner. Health care organizations which departmentalize by function place together specialists with the same kind of education, background, equipment, and facility needs. Under arrangements such as these, the supervisor will be concerned with only one form of patient care as well as one type of health care professional. The primary advantage of functional departmentalization is that it allows a better coordination of services and places together a group of professionals with similar interests. For this reason, it is one of the most widely used methods of organizing in a health care facility.

By Product

In the industrial sector of the economy, the principle of product departmentalization is quite common. Here, a specific product is produced as a relatively independent unit within the organization. A company like Chrysler Corporation, for example, may produce two products: automobiles and trucks. The two separate products would require separate divisions for engineering, design, supplies, equipment, and for the ordering of resources. The two divisions would be operated without any influence from one another but would still be a part of the "whole" of Chrysler Corporation.

In health care, product departmentalization is not very common. Dividing a hospital into "products" would involve individual products such as radiology, surgery, and intensive care. Each of these departments would need its own supervisor of medical records, supervisor of dietary, supervisor of nursing and all the other services required by an individual department. Each product department would also have its own director who would be in charge of all services within the department.

Organizing a hospital by product will result in a profound duplication of effort. Instead of a single director of physical therapy, there would be as many directors of physical therapy as there are departments who utilize the services. Coordination of services becomes almost impossible. Inability to coordinate services is the primary reason why product departmentalization is not applicable to most health care settings.

By Territory

Another way to departmentalize is to designate a specific area where a segment of the population requires health care services but are widely dispersed or difficult to reach. There may, for example, be certain geographical considerations which may limit health care services being provided to those patients who really need them. Hospitals are increasingly investigating the establishment of home health agencies to provide health care services to those patients in rural areas who cannot travel to the institution in order to obtain health care. Providing health care services in this manner promotes organizational goodwill in the community and helps to ensure patients will return to the hospital for outpatient procedures and emergency care.

By Customer

Customer departmentalization is often seen in those health care centers who attempt to satisfy the needs of both inpatients and outpatients. Increasingly, hospitals are establishing outpatient surgery centers to accommodate the particular needs of those patients who do not require hospital admission following surgery. Surgery for cataracts, as well as many types of orthopaedic surgery, are now performed on a one-day, non-admission basis. Some hospital physical therapy departments and private practitioners have established evening and weekend hours to accommodate those patients who cannot attend regularly scheduled sessions. Those facilities who offer back school programs do so to accommodate the needs of a particular group of patients. Attempting to attract a particular customer is one way for a facility to broaden the health care service they offer to a community and increase their profitability.

By Process and Equipment

Departmentalization by process and equipment is very similar to departmentalization by function. All activities involving certain types of equipment or specialized technical considerations may be grouped together. For example, a neurologist may request a patient with symptoms of quadricep weakness bilaterally to have an isokinetic test to ascertain if there is such a problem. Even though the doctor did not specifically order the physical therapy department to perform the test, it would most likely be conducted by a physical therapist. A physical therapy department may be departmentalized by both function and equipment, since much of the equipment used in patient care is sophisticated and can be used on a variety of patient illnesses and disorders.

By Time

To some extent, any hospital which provides health care on a continual basis must departmentalize by time. The department of nursing is often divided into day, afternoon, and night shifts. Offering health care services on a 24-hour-a-day basis is a requirement for most health care settings. It does, however, present potential problems in coordinating patient services and in personnel management. Instances arise where messages are not forwarded and physician orders are not implemented. This is especially true when one shift is preparing to leave work while another is just beginning. A physical therapy department may partially departmentalize by time if health services are offered from 7:00 A.M. to 7:00 or 8:00 P.M. Here, some personnel may arrive early and leave around 3:30 P.M. while others may arrive later and provide coverage until closing.

Staffing

In all health care organizations it is the manager's responsibility to recruit human resources to meet the employment needs of the institution. Staffing is the process by which a health care manager seeks qualified individuals to fill the various positions within the department. Once the department has been organized and duties have been assigned, individuals must be located to provide services which will allow the department and organization to meet planned objectives and goals. For the physical therapy supervisor, staffing includes the selection, training, appraisal and development of personnel throughout the various stages of their professional careers.

Performing the staffing function is a continuous activity for a health care supervisor. It is mistakenly assumed that the staffing function is only performed when opening a new department. A more accurate assessment is to think of the staffing function as a situation where the supervisor is placed in charge of an established physical therapy department with a group of employees already present. Even though the employees are present, sooner or later personnel changes will take place. It is therefore the supervisor's responsibility to make sure there is a continual supply of well-trained individuals to fill employment positions as they become available.

Influencing

Influencing is the health care managerial function which evokes action from personnel to accomplish the organization's objectives and goals. Often referred to as motivating, directing and actuating, the function has many dimensions. Some of these dimensions include employee morale and satisfaction, worker productivity and leadership as well as communication. When the supervisor performs the managerial function of influencing, he or she attempts to create a climate which is conducive to employee satisfaction while at the same time achieving the objectives and goals of the organization.

Every physical therapy supervisor must be aware of the multiple of human interactions which occur within the department. Additionally, the supervisor must be aware of the ways in which influence can be exerted upon them to improve the quality of care provided. The influencing function is not only a means for getting work done but also for developing employees to their fullest potential. A supervisor can have a profound effect upon an employee by teaching and guiding the individual to a better understanding of the organization. Properly performing the influencing function can build an effective work force by inspiring each individual to perform as though he or she were working for themselves. The health care manager has the ultimate responsibility for instilling motivation within the employee to perform enthusiastically while at the same time helping the individual to obtain personal satisfaction from the job.

Controlling

The managerial function of controlling determines whether organizational and departmental objectives and goals have been achieved. When an organization plans to achieve certain outcomes there must be a check to determine whether the results obtained meet with the preestablished criteria. Therefore, the managerial function of controlling is tied very closely to the managerial function of planning. Whenever objectives and goals are not met, corrective action must be taken to get the organization or individual department back on the right course. Planning decisions ultimately affect the control methods that are established. In the same fashion, the control process affects an organization's current and future plans.

Many health care managers see the controlling function as something which is done after the fact. This is often because problems are not discovered until after a mistake has been made. For the physical therapist as a health care supervisor, controlling is not something which is to be done after the fact but rather a managerial function which helps to incorporate the other managerial functions. Controlling is, therefore, interrelated to the managerial functions of planning, organizing, staffing, and influencing. The better each one of these functions are performed, the more successful the controlling function will be.

Controlling provides management in the organization with an opportunity to continually look to the future. When standards have been set, based upon past events, management can anticipate future sources of deviation and make the necessary corrections to avoid problems. Without exercising control, a manager cannot be performing all aspects of a job. The health care manager must assign employees tasks and delegate authority and responsibility for task accomplishment. He or she must then exercise control to see that tasks are carried out according to the predetermined standards.

The eventual success of the physical therapy department, and the level of care provided to the patient, depends upon the degree of difference between what an employee should do and what has been done. When the supervisor sets a standard of performance, there must be a continual check of performance. This can be accomplished by way of observation, the use of reports, the computation of statistical data, or other similar methods. Each of these tools will be of assistance in evaluating what has been accomplished and additional actions that may be needed to bring about full compliance.

APPLYING THE MANAGERIAL FUNCTIONS

The five managerial functions are performed by all managers regardless of their position within the health care organization. The amount of time spent and the managerial effort applied to each function will depend upon the position of the supervisor within the health care organization. Top administrators will spend little time in direct employee supervision. They will be more concerned with planning and organizing the facility along with a careful eye to future events. The supervisor of a physical therapy department will, on the other hand, be more concerned with the managerial functions of staffing, influencing, and controlling.

The five functions blend together in a continuous process as is demonstrated in Figure 1-7. There is no clear demarcation indicating where a manager will end one function and begin another. A health care manager's time and effort spent on each function will depend on circumstances which will vary on a daily basis. One thing is for certain: no health care manager can organize, staff, control, or influence without plans. Therefore, the planning function must take priority in any health care organization. The physical therapist who plans decides in advance which courses are to be followed and what policies, procedures, and methods are to be used. Even the smallest of physical therapy departments must use physical and human resources in an efficient manner. As a supervisor, planning will allow you to bring out the best in each of your health care employees—the most valuable resources you have.

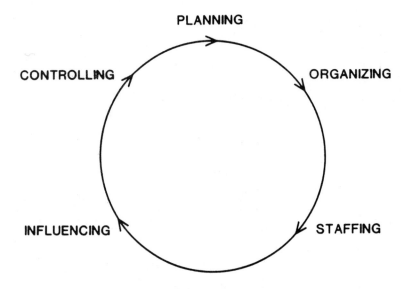

THE MANAGERIAL FUNCTIONS

Figure 1-7.

MANAGING PROFESSIONAL EMPLOYEES

The modern health care environment has, within the past twenty years, been experiencing a rapid increase in the amount of specialization. This is well evidenced in the profession of physical therapy, where sub-speciality certification is now a reality. The development of sub-specialities is due in part to the fact there is now too much to learn to allow anyone to claim a complete understanding of the entire field of physical therapy. It is for this reason medical doctors specialize in any number of fields (neurology, pediatrics, rheumatology, etc.) upon graduation from medical school.

As is well known, physicians, physical therapists, and attorneys have long practiced their professions in groups. Hospitals and rehabilitation centers also group similar health care professions into one department or area. Practicing a profession in a group provides the opportunity for a number of related specialists to offer a broader range of health care services in one location. The advantage to the patient is that a greater degree of skill can be applied to the health care problem than if each health care member practiced independently. In other words, grouping trained health care professionals together can result in better patient care.

Bringing together a group of health care professionals with similar interests and desires can stimulate an environment that produces high-quality patient care. At the same time, managing a group of professionals, such as physical therapists, can present a health care manager with many unique management problems. Understanding how to manage professionals begins with an appreciation of some of the intriguing characteristics and issues of managing professional employees.

CHARACTERISTICS OF PROFESSIONAL EMPLOYEES

There are two factors which separate professional employees, such as a physical therapist, from other non-professional health care providers in an organization. One factor has to do with the value they represent to the health care organization. The other has to do with the unique characteristics which professional employees share that separate them from other non-professional organizational members.

For a health care organization, whether it be a hospital or a private office, the physical therapist represents an extremely valuable asset. Their value as a professional is derived from two sources. First, the health care organization relies on the professional to provide quality patient care. Quality patient care is obtained from the individual member's professional commitment to excellence. New ideas, treatment methods, and advances in patient rehabilitation all originate from the commitment of the professional. The financial investment to retain the health care professional may be costly to the employer, but it is often rewarded through the continual stream of new ideas and approaches to the rehabilitation of patients.

The second source of value to the health care organization comes from the expert knowledge the professional brings to the job. There are increasing demands placed on the physical therapist through intensive educational processes and examinations which the individual must complete in order to gain professional standing as a physical therapist. The physical therapist, as a highly trained member of the health care organization, can exercise these skills to the benefit of not only patients but also non-professional employees and the local community. Many individuals and organizations, outside of the immediate employment environment, can benefit from the expert knowledge the physical therapist has to offer.

CHARACTERISTICS OF THE PHYSICAL THERAPIST AS A PROFESSIONAL

Individuals who enter the profession of physical therapy often share a similar set of unique personality characteristics. Some of these characteristics, such as a genuine concern for people, seem quite obvious. Others make a generalized assumption but still tend to refer to the individual as a highly dedicated health care professional. The following list of characteristics clearly establish the profession of physical therapy as a leader in providing health care services:

- The physical therapist has invested heavily in terms of time and energy in order to prepare themselves for the profession.
- There are a large number of potential employers for both the new graduate and the established professional. If employment in one health care organization does not meet with satisfaction, the physical therapist will likely seek employment elsewhere.
- The profession of physical therapy is essentially intellectually and theoretically based.
- The profession is bound by a service orientation. Above all, the professional is not concerned with self-interest but rather the welfare of the patient.
- The profession of physical therapy is not standardized. The approach to patient care recognizes each individual as unique.
- The health care services provided by the physical therapist are presumed to be dependent upon the patient's needs and not on their ability to pay.
- The relationship between the patient and the physical therapist is based on trust and respect for the individual's dignity.

- As professionals, physical therapists often have a very strong loyalty and identity with the profession. These loyalties may, in some instances, be in direct conflict with the employing organization's ideas concerning loyalty and ethics.
- The profession of physical therapy, and its educational institutions, are guided by a professional association. The professional association serves to protect and inform its members as well as maintain the highest of professional standards in health care.
- As a professional, the physical therapist is expected to behave in an appropriate manner, remaining emotionally detatched, to ensure all patient health care decisions are based strictly on medical-technical grounds.

Each of these characteristics clearly identifies the physical therapist as a health care professional. As a professional, the physical therapist will desire to only work in facilities which recognize their importance to the organization. Supervising health care professionals can be a challenging task requiring knowledge about the proper methods to use to help ensure member satisfaction.

SUPERVISING THE PHYSICAL THERAPIST AS A PROFESSIONAL EMPLOYEE

An important consideration for maintaining job satisfaction among physical therapists, regardless of the health care setting, is the proper selection of a department manager. The person who occupies the supervisory position will be responsible for establishing the environment which is conducive to the provision of quality patient care. In the modern health care environment, the physical therapy supervisor must realize the ever-increasing degree to which the staff physical therapist, as a member of the organization, will exercise authority in decisions concerning patient care and department operation.

The physical therapist has a well-recognized set of specialized skills and abilities and, as such, enjoys a degree of influence in the organization. This degree of influence will extend beyond just direct patient care to also include the ability to influence the members of the hospital's administration and members of the medical community. The ability to exercise informal influence can create problems for the director of physical therapy, especially when professional employees bypass their supervisor to discuss departmental matters with members of the hospital's top management.

It is, therefore, essential that the supervisor of physical therapy exercise a great deal of flexability in departmental operations. Supervising the professional must include recognition of the fact that they are influenced by not only the supervisor but also by professional considerations and relations with those outside the department. The supervisor who makes an active effort to maintain open lines of communication with professional employees, reduces the chances of personnel and professional problems being carried outside the department for eventual resolution.

JOB PREFERENCES FOR THE PHYSICAL THERAPIST

Physical therapists place a high priority on patient treatment assignments that are both challenging and sufficiently stimulating to provide them with a sense of achievement. The therapist often strives to obtain outstanding results from patient care and is willing to work hard to accomplish these goals. Increasingly, the professional is seeking the opportunity to further personal discretion in providing patient care. To help in achieving these goals, many professionals are demanding the most modern and up-to-date departmental environments in which to work. To meet these requirements often involves prerequisites such as the availability of specialized equipment, freedom in scheduling certain patient treatment regimes as well as a reduction in many of the routine departmental and patient treatment tasks.

To be an effective health care supervisor requires a thorough understanding of individual preferences within the department. The assignment of a patient to a particular therapist should always consider the health care professional's abilities and interests. The matching of a patient to a therapist should remain consistent with the objectives and goals of the health care organization. Some physical therapists prefer to work alone and uninterrupted, while others prefer the stimulation that a group of health care professionals can provide. Whenever possible, the structure and operation of the department should be arranged to accommodate the therapist's individual preferences rather than running counter to them.

To encourage creativity in patient care, the supervisor should provide an environment that is open and permissive. This can only be accomplished by establishing a climate in which the criticism of ideas by both professional and non-professional employees is avoided and judgment is withheld. The supervisor should also allow the departments' professional employees the opportunity to engage in conversations with one another without interruption. This can be accomplished by conducting weekly meetings between the management of the department and the staff physical therapists and physical therapy assistants. Meetings such as these provide professional interaction and give each member an opportunity to air grievances and opinions.

PROFESSIONAL REWARDS ISSUES

Health care professionals with unique or specialized training may present substantial problems for a supervisor who desires to provide individual rewards. In many areas of business, the individual's traditional promotional path involves the transition from technical proficiency in job performance to a managerial or administrative assignment. This same career path is also available to the physical therapist who has the desire and motivation to accept a managerial position.

In health care, however, the promotional path may become a dilemma for the physical therapist who is highly skilled in their area of expertise, enjoys practicing the profession but has absolutely no aspirations towards health care management. When pressured, they may eventually assume a managerial position but will ultimately become dissatisfied with the additional responsibility and job requirements.

When presented with situations such as these, the health care manager must consider special promotional paths for the physical therapist who is at this stage of a career. In many hospital settings, for example, opportunities for nurses to be promoted have been divided into two separate paths: one managerial and the other clinical. Establishing a clinical position makes it possible for a nurse with no managerial interests to earn increases in pay and rise within the organization through the continual development of professional skills. Career paths such as these have also been developed for the physical therapist. Those professionals who have no interest in health care management may seek increased professional rewards through the clinical supervision of physical therapy students. Still other physical therapists find diversity in patient care by treating patients at hospital bedside when the individual's medical condition prevents them from being treated in the physical therapy department.

Health care managers who create parallel paths of career advancement, one managerial and the other based on specialized skills and interests, can reduce the likelihood of employee frustration. To implement a structure such as this may require the rule "no one should make more money than the department director" be discarded. The longstanding concern that the director be the most highly paid individual may not be appropriate if the development of a specialized program requires the unique abilities of one highly trained individual.

The salary offered to attract a professional to an organization is also a critical factor. Many physical therapists are initially attracted to a facility by the promise of a high salary. High salaries must be offered to attract competent, skilled and energetic health care professionals. The consequence of offering a high salary is that future raises may seem incrementally small. This perception can result in job dissatisfaction for the professional employee. To help in the prevention of this problem, the organization can encourage further professional development through subsidizing attendance at professional meetings. Recognition can also be provided to those physical therapists who actively engage in research projects concerning patient treatment or develop ways to improve efficiency and productivity within the department.

HEALTH CARE MANAGEMENT—THE EFFICIENT COMBINATION OF KNOWLEDGE AND EXPERIENCE

No one book on health care management can teach you everything that is needed to become an effective health care manager and ensure your department or practice provides high-quality patient care. To become the best health care manager possible, you must have personal ability, desire, and a thorough understanding of the necessary management skills. One of the best ways to become a skilled supervisor is to work with an established health care manager who is in a position of responsibility. Much can be learned by analyzing what a proven leader does, how he or she does it, and what results are obtained.

Throughout your professional career as a physical therapist you will undoubtedly work with both good and bad health care managers. You will quickly observe that it is much easier to learn from a good manager than it is to learn from a poor one. This is not to say that you cannot learn a number of things from a poor one; it is simply more important to learn what to do than what not to do.

A good health care manager not only takes pride in the quality of health care provided but also has a desire to interact with and provide pleasant surroundings for fellow health care professionals. For that reason, every prospective employment position should be evaluated not only from the standpoint of professional rewards but from the aspect of who will be your immediate supervisor. Putting your own management skills to work can greatly be enhanced by a supervisor who actively takes an interest in your career and allows you to assume a leadership role in the health care organization.

The principles and skills discussed in this book can, of course, be learned. Knowing and understanding how to properly motivate employees is vital to the performance of your department. None of the skills which are contained within this book can be learned overnight. The only way to become a successful supervisor is to work hard at properly applying the principles of management to your department or practice situation. You undoubtedly will make mistakes, but you can learn from those mistakes. The effort you apply to increasing your managerial competence will ultimately pay handsome rewards. Before long, you will be able to prevent many of the difficulties which make a supervisory position a burden instead of a challenging and satisfying career.

REFERENCES

1. "The Corporate Elite," Business Week, October 21, 1988, p. 198.
2. "Grays On The Go," Time, February 22, 1988, p. 70.
3. Adapted from Robert Katz, "Skills of an Effective Administrator," Harvard Business Review, September–October 1974, pp. 90–102.
4. Henri Fayol, Industrial and General Administration, trans. J. A. Coubrough (Geneva: International Management Institute, 1929).

Chapter Two

THE HEALTH CARE ORGANIZATION
AS A SYSTEM

The hospital, rehabilitation center, nursing home and private practice physical therapy center are all examples of systems. Although each of these organizations is separate from one another, each is still, in part, dependent upon one another. Recognizing any health care organization as a system requires the manager look beyond single-cause thinking. General systems theory recognizes each of these independent parts as making up the whole, which is in turn interdependent within the external environment.[1]

Utilizing general systems thinking encourages the health care manager to look beyond the cause-and-effect relationships that occur in a physical therapy department. The health care manager should not look at just a single cause of a problem but instead at the broader number of possibilities. For instance, the director of physical therapy may recognize that employees are willing to join the organization, report satisfaction with employment, but leave the organization after six months to one year. Utilizing systems theory the manager should look beyond the department for possible reasons for the high turnover. There may be other factors within and outside of the organization which are contributing to the problem.

Examining the organization from a systems perspective forces the manager to abandon the flat two-dimensional organizational chart such as the one depicted in Figure 2-1. The organizational chart is a convenient model that helps the members of the organization visualize the complicated relationships which are in existence. In the modern health care environment it would probably be more accurate to portray the health care organization with a mobile instead of with a flat two-dimensional chart. Whenever you touch one part of a mobile, the remaining parts will react to the contact in some fashion. Movement will occur in some or all parts of the mobile, even though the changes in position are not instaneous but instead occur over time. The same is true in a hospital physical therapy department. A change instituted by a member of top management, a medical doctor, or a staff member can change other parts of the organization and potentially redirect its future.

BASIC REQUIREMENTS OF SYSTEMS THINKING

All health care professionals are at least partially familiar with the concept of systems theory. We often speak of the respiratory system, circulatory system and other systems within the human body. In management it is not uncommon to hear terms such as *management information systems* or *communication systems.* The word system is appropriate in health care management because it conveys the idea that each of the parts of an organization interact with one another. A system, as such, is recognized as an organized group of parts, people and equipment that act as a complex whole. There is an inherent sense of interdependency.

Originally developed as part of engineering operations and production management, systems theory has increasingly become recognized as part of the health care system. There is a tremendous amount of interdependency among the various providers in the health care environ-

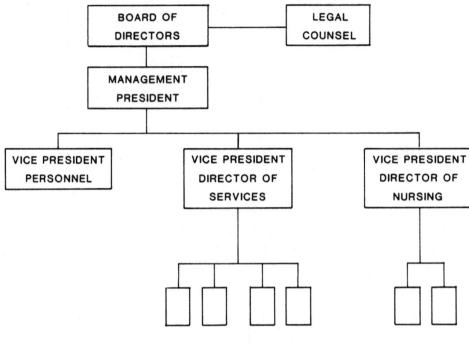

Figure 2-1.

ment. In a hospital, if a change is implemented in one aspect of operation, it is likely to have a ripple effect on the remainder of the organization. The same is true in patient care. If a medical doctor orders a set of tests be performed on a patient, all other services involved with the diagnosis and treatment of that patient will be at least partially influenced by the test results.

Another important aspect of general systems theory is the idea of "wholism." The idea behind wholism is that an organization as a system should be recognized as a functioning whole. Any proposed change should be considered from the standpoint of its potential impact on the organization's overall performance. An administrator's proposal, for example, to start a cardiac rehabilitation unit must take into consideration the impact such a unit will have on the rest of the organization. The unit will undoubtedly require substantial financial backing in order to recruit and retain personnel. If the physical therapy department is to be involved, the director of the department will require additional personnel, department space, and a financial commitment from the organization. The concept of systems theory forces the administrator and the department director to consider the impact of change at all levels, not just in one department.

Synergism is another important concept in the theory of general systems. Synergism is the working together of all the interactive parts of the organization. When the various departments work together as one, the effect will be far greater than the outcome produced when each acts independently. A rehabilitative group consisting of a speech therapist, occupational therapist, and a physical therapist can accomplish more working closely together in providing patient care services than if each acted independently without consultation. The same is true when the remaining departments of the organization work together.

Subsystems: Parts of the Total System

When analyzing a health care organization it will soon become readily apparent that the system is made up of a number of subsystems. A subsystem is a small group, department, or speciality area within a larger system. They are classified as smaller systems within the total system of the organization. An example of a subsystem can be found by examining the department of nursing in a hospital. Within the department of nursing there are smaller departments for nurses who specialize in orthopaedics, neurology, oncology, pediatrics, and many other areas. Each of these subsystems are parts of the total system of nursing in the organization.

Boundaries for systems can be established by top management in the organization. The department of physical therapy in a university can be considered a subsystem in the field of allied health. Within the department of physical therapy, subsystems can be identified such as the undergraduate, graduate and the postgraduate programs. For purposes of analysis, subsystems can be divided as needed in order to isolate the area to be examined. Figure 2-2 further demonstrates the differences between systems and subsystems.

The Workings of the System

In order to function properly, a system requires inputs, a transformation process, and outputs. A health care organization's inputs are the resources it applies to providing patient care services. These resources can include labor, information, energy, and materials. The resources and inputs are provided by the external environment or by one of the subsystems

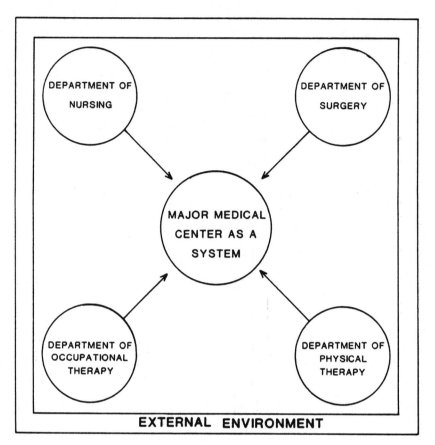

Figure 2-2.

within the health care organization (Figure 2-3). A patient who arrives at the emergency room, for example, will require a number of inputs in order to assess the severity of the condition. The patient may require extensive labor from emergency-room physicians, nurses, and x-ray technologists. Each will provide valuable inputs that enable decisions to be made concerning the severity of the injury.

The activities performed within the health care organization serve to transform the inputs into outputs. In the case of the patient who arrived in the emergency room, surgery may be required to transform the person to the level they were before the accident. After surgery, the patient will require nursing services and possibly the care provided by a physical therapist.

An output is the final product produced by the efforts of all of those involved in the transformation process. The output of the hypothetical

THE HOSPITAL

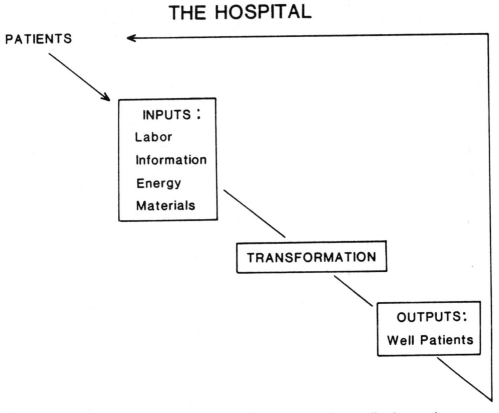

Patients enter the system, receive care, and are discharged from the hospital, to hopefully return again if additional services are required.

Figure 2-3.

emergency-room patient would be for the person to leave the hospital and return to his or her previous environment. The physical therapist's final discharge of the patient from rehabilitative services is also considered an output.

Properly considered the input-transformation-output process is made up of six steps. They are:

1) Determination of the type and quality of inputs.
2) Determination of the sources of inputs.
3) Implementing the transformation process.
4) Determination of an acceptable level of output.
5) Determination of the subsystems used in the output process.
6) Establishing a network of feedback.

To develop a thorough understanding of the input-transformation-output process of systems theory, refer to Figure 2-4 while considering the role a trauma team will play in the following six steps:

1) *Determination of the type and quantity of inputs.* A hospital that desires to establish itself as a trauma center does so in order to be recognized as a leader in providing a comprehensive set of health care services. Members of the trauma team are chosen based on their expertise in treating severely injured persons who arrive for emergency care. Members chosen to head the trauma team would include a neurosurgeon, orthopaedic surgeon, general surgeon, cardiovascular surgeon, anesthesiologist, and many other highly trained professionals. As members of the team they would be on call 24 hours a day and remain easily accessible for emergency situations.

2) *Determination of the sources of inputs.* The individuals recruited to become members of the team would require special qualifications. Their educational backgrounds should include a wide variety of emergency-room experience and in-depth surgical training.

3) *Implementing the transformation process.* The process of establishing a trauma team requires an organization give careful consideration to an understanding of the conditions under which members would be called to the hospital. Implementing the transformation process should also include the appointment of a medical director to over-see its operation and act upon requests made by trauma team members.

4) *Determination of an acceptable level of outputs.* Trauma team members must have the responsibility and authority to see a patient gets whatever is needed in life-or-death situations. For example, it may be determined that a child suffering from third-degree burns would be better off transferred to a facility which specializes in treatment of acutely injured children. The team must have the authority to arrange for special transportation and arrive at a consensus as to how soon the child must be transferred.

5) *Determination of the subsystems used in the output process.* Highly traumatized individuals often require a number of skilled health care professionals to assist them through the rehabilitation process. Trauma team members will be responsible for deciding which services a patient will require throughout the recovery process.

Some of the most common services utilized will include physical therapy, occupational therapy, respiratory therapy and social services.

6) *The feedback process.* A highly skilled group of professionals, such as a trauma team, must have a well-developed system of feedback. The members must know which areas need to be improved and changed. Feedback should be solicited from fellow team members, patients, allied health care professionals, and from the external environment. Only through direct discussions of treatment results can members ascertain how performance can be improved.

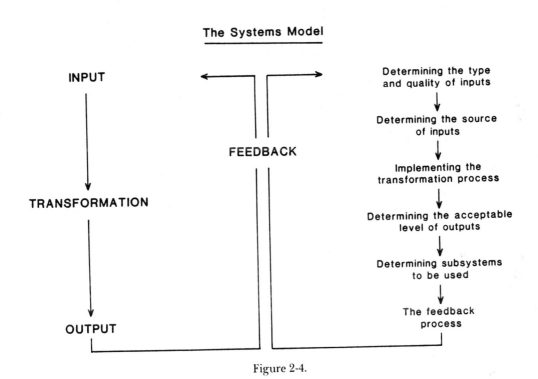

Figure 2-4.

The trauma team example provides an outline of how systems theory works in the health care organization as well as demonstrating the importance of feedback. No department, private practice, or health care organization can effectively improve the services it offers without understanding how the services are perceived by patients. Feedback completes the systems theory loop and allows the organization to make the necessary changes for continued survival.

Open and Closed Systems

The analysis of a health care organization as a system must consider the possibility that it can be viewed as either an open or closed system. An open system is one which continually interacts with the external environment. It is part of the environment and is acted upon by the environment. A closed system is one which does not interact with its environment. A person who examines an organization from the closed-system perspective looks solely at the organization and does not consider the effects of the external environment on the organization.

Biological systems, such as plants, are considered open systems. The plant relies specifically upon the external environment for a continual supply of food, water, soil, and carbon dioxide. It also acts upon the environment by producing seeds to expand its number and by producing oxygen for animal and human consumption. As such, very few systems can be considered closed.

It may be possible to temporarily consider a system as closed if performing an in-depth organizational analysis. Systems cannot, however, remain closed for long without eventually suffering from entrophy. An organization which suffers from entrophy expends more energy than it is able to take in from the external environment.

A physical therapist who first enters private practice is likely to become familar with the concept of entrophy. Initially, the physical therapist may see a large volume of patients but collect little in monies for the services provided. In other words, energy in the form of work is going out, but the financial rewards are not immediately ascertainable. Ideally, the physical therapist will attempt to achieve the state of negative entrophy. In the coming months he or she will hope to take in as much or more energy than is expended. In other words, the goal is to keep the system from deteriorating or going bankrupt. The system deteriorates when salaries, rent, light, and water bills cannot be paid.

Health care organizations of all types are considered open systems. A health care organization acts upon and is acted upon by a number of elements in the external environment. Health care managers who adopt closed-systems thinking are unrealistic about their particular organization's role in society. Organizations and managers who fail to recognize the influence provided by the external environment will soon be overwhelmed by organizations who recognize its importance.

Static and Dynamic Systems

Health care organizations can also be considered either static or dynamic systems. A system which is considered static is one in which little or no change takes place. The dynamic system is one in which changes do occur over a period of time. A chair is a good example of a static system, since it consists of a seat, back, and four legs and demonstrates very little change over time. Most health care organizations are considered dynamic systems because of the rate and degree of change which is occurring in the health care industry. One of the more recent factors influencing the American health care system is the federal government's implementation of diagnostically related groups, or DRG's.

On April 1, 1983, Congress passed legislation enacting the Medicare Prospective Payment System. The intent of the legislation was to fix the per-case payment rates for each of 468 diagnosis-related groups into which a patient could be classified. The legislation became a mechanism for transferring the risk from payer to provider. No longer would a hospital get paid more for having a patient stay longer. Under the per-case payment system, Medicare pays the hospital a fixed price for a service. The DRG system has forced hospitals to be more cost effective and know what the exact cost is for a particular set of health care services. If, for example, Medicare recognizes a hospital stay of 14 days for a total hip replacement, it would not be cost effective for the hospital to allow the patient to stay 21 days. The hospital will receive the same amount of money regardless of the patient's length of stay.

The implementation of the prospective payment system has had a profound effect on hospitals and medicine. Since its implementation, hospital occupancy rates have decreased, affecting both hospitals and doctors. A medical doctor who has admitting priviledges at several hospitals may be encouraged to admit patients at one hospital over another. Once the physician has admitted the patient, the practitioner will then be encouraged to discharge the patient at the earliest possible convenience.

To date, diagnostic-related groups do not apply to professional changes such as physician office visits. There is the possibility that the Health Care Financing Administration may want to extend the concept to include physician fees. If this occurs, the physician who sees a patient in a private office would only receive a fixed dollar amount for the diagnosis and treatment of a disease or ailment. The fixed-fee system would apply no matter how many times the physician needed to see the patient.

The external environment is also a dynamic place for the physical therapist. The American Physical Therapy Association strongly supports the Ethics in Patient Referrals Act of 1989 (H.R. 939).[2] The idea behind the proposed legislation is that a referring doctor should not be permitted to profit directly or indirectly from the act of prescribing services that Medicare will reimburse. The proposed legislation prohibits a physician from referring a patient for a Medicare-covered service to a provider if the physician or an immediate family member has an ownership or investment interest in the provider or other compensation arrangement. If passed, the bill will be one step towards further enhancing the therapist's ability to practice the profession without physician influence.

THE IMPORTANCE OF THE EXTERNAL ENVIRONMENT

Forces external to the organization were first incorporated into management thought during the late 1950s. The recognition of the importance of the external environment is one of the major contributions of the systems approach to management. The idea stressed the need for managers to view their organization as a mixture of interrelated parts that intertwine with the outside world. Today, the changes in health care have made it more important than ever to consider the external environment. As has been stated by Alvar Elbing, "The external environment of an organization is a subject of increasing challenge for today's managers. In fact, the managers of society's major organizations; business, education, and government have been forced by recent events to place an increasing focus on a rapidly changing environment and its effect on the internal organization."[3]

A health care professional who desires to adopt the view of the external environment as an open system cannot possibly consider all of the influencing factors. Only those which are of relative importance can be considered. Gerald Bell believes, "An organization's external environment consists of those things outside the organization such as customers, competitors, government, financial firms, and labor pools that are relevent to an organization's operations."[4] A number of factors influence the operation of a health care organization. Some have a far greater impact on the organization than others. Two forces are closely linked with understanding systems theory as it applies to the external environment. The forces are identified as either direct action or indirect action environmental variables.

Those variables considered part of the direct action environment will directly affect, or are affected by, the operation of the health care organization. Factors included would be suppliers, laws, patients, competitors and labor unions. Those factors in the indirect action environment may not directly influence the organization and its operations, but they must, nevertheless, be considered as influential. Factors relevent in the indirect action environment include the economy, medical technology, sociocultural variables and political developments.

The physical therapist aspiring to own a private practice will be directly affected by the actions of medical doctors, the local hospital, chiropractors, osteopaths, and other physical therapists in private practice. The practitioner must remain attuned to changes in the local community in order to gain a competitive edge. The reactions and actions of some of these professional groups will undoubtedly, directly or indirectly, influence the growth and ultimate survival of the practice.

Characteristics of the Environment

Medical professionals historically give most of their attention to their own medical practice, economic situation, and their immediate professional environment. To become a leader in the health care profession, the practitioner must now give greater attention to the changes in human values, social values, political movements, and to the legal aspects of practice. Emery and Trist believe that there is increasing turbulence in the external environment. "Managers can no longer consider each environmental factor independently. Managers today must give greater consideration to the factors of environmental complexity, volatility and uncertainty.[5]"

The more complex the environment, the more likely changes can be expected. Medical care is growing rapidly in the United States due in part to the sophisticated advances in technology. The field is also growing with an increased number of specialists whose responsibility is only one small aspect of patient care. If the present trends in health care continue as they are, the generalist will undoubtedly become more and more a thing of the past.

Volatility is the rate at which an organization's environment is changing.

Researchers in management are increasingly recognizing the rate at which the environment of the contemporary organization is changing. Changes are occurring in the profession of physical therapy due in part to the use of the computer and to the rapidly expanding base of medical knowledge. The profession of physical therapy is increasingly recognized as volatile because of the rapid rate the profession is changing. The profession recently established speciality areas and is becoming more diverse in the services it offers to patients.

Environmental uncertainty is the degree to which the environment moves from one that is stable and simple to one which is dynamic and complex. For hospitals, the environment has increasingly become more complex. Many hospitals are expanding from the traditional concepts of patient care into more diverse areas. Hospitals are expanding the delivery of their services into such areas as ambulatory clinics, substance abuse and detoxification centers, nursing home care, hospices and home health agencies. The development of these services is often in direct response to the federal government's implementation of the diagnostic-related groups system of hospital reimbursement. Hospitals, in order to be cost effective, must try to limit the length of stay for the patient. In response to this requirement, many are providing outpatient services to gain additional profitability.

The Direct Action Environment

The direct action environment consists of those consumers, government agencies, competitors, suppliers and laws which directly influence how the organization operates. Each of these is recognized as specific to a given organization but will undoubtedly change in number and composition over time.

Suppliers

The systems concept encourages the health care manager to view the organization as one which transforms inputs into outputs. In either the hospital-based physical therapy department or in private practice the major source of inputs will be materials, energy, capital, and labor. The relationship between the health care organization and the network of suppliers is one of the best examples of how the external environment can affect the hospital and the private office. If the director of physical therapy is unable to obtain the essential inputs that are required to achieve objectives, the quality and quantity of care delivered to the patient will deteriorate. One of the greatest problems facing the director of a department is that of obtaining labor. Nationally, it has been estimated that the demand for physical therapists will continue to rise past the year 2000. The supply of labor and how it can be attracted to an organization will be an important issue for years to come.

Laws and Government Agencies

The laws and government agencies who oversee them undoubtedly influence how health care is practiced in the United States. All health care institutions, and the individuals who own or operate them, are subject to federal and state laws regarding how they should be managed. Medicare, which began on July 1, 1966, has a profound influence on how many of the health care services are delivered in this country.

Medicare consists of two complementary programs which are available to those age 65 years and older. Medicare Part A covers primarily inpatient hospitalization but will also cover care delivered in certain long-term skilled nursing facilities or in the patient's home. The supplemental medical insurance, known as Medicare Part B, covers physician services, hospital outpatient services, and care provided by home health agencies.

Medicaid, also established in 1966, is a joint venture between the federal government and the individual states. The program is specifically designed to meet the needs of the poor. Each of the fifty states administers its own program and defines eligibility requirements and covered services. Although the federal government does establish minimum standards for individual eligibility, its primary role is one of matching state funds. Coverage provided under Medicaid includes:

1) Inpatient and outpatient hospital care.
2) Early and periodic screening and diagnostic testing.
3) Laboratory and x-ray services.
4) Care in a skilled nursing facility.
5) Home health services.
6) Family planning services.
7) Physician services.

Eligibility for Medicaid varies widely across states, with some having eligibility standards below the federal poverty line while others have expanded eligibility to include other medically needy groups.[6]

Medicare and Medicaid have greatly influenced how health care services are provided in the United States. Current estimates indicate the federal government pays for approximately 40 percent of all health care expenditures. Due to the increasing budget deficits at the federal level it is likely legislation will continue to be implemented, which further shifts the burden of payment toward the consumer.

Customers

The health care requirements of the consumer strongly influence which services are available and at what price. Increasingly, however, price is becoming more of a concern for the consumer and for many of major insurers of health care. Medical expenses are outpacing the consumer price index. The present annual health care bill now exceeds $500 billion and may represent as much as 15 percent of the gross national product by the year 2000.[7]

As a result of the growing costs for health care, many insurers are looking for ways to reduce their out-of-pocket costs. Small business owners have begun reducing the health care benefits they offer or have stopped offering health care plans entirely. Health care expenditures have increased at an average annual rate of 10.4 percent during the period from 1950 to 1985. Since that time, the United States has gone from spending about $1 billion per year for health care to more than $1 billion per day by 1985.[8]

Competitors

Competition has never been greater than it is now for the health care dollar. In 1958, medical schools in the United States were graduating approximately 6,861 students each year. At that time, the physician/population ratio was only 144 physicians per 100,000 population. Presently, there are 127 United States medical schools graduating 16,000 doctors per year. The ratio is estimated at 200 physicians per 100,000 of population. The physician/population ratio is growing three times faster than the general population.[9]

The 1980 Graduate Medical Educational National Advisory Committee (GMENAC) predicted that if medical schools continue to graduate classes at the present size there will be an oversupply of approximately 70,000 doctors by the year 1990.[10] Growing numbers of physicians will have a substantial influence on the American health care system. General economic theory and common sense would argue that if the number of physicians increase, their net income will fall which will discourage others from entering the profession. Some researchers believe, however, that a growth in the number of physicians results in a disproportionate increase in the number of health care expenditures. In other words, the more doctors, the more hospital admissions, the more tests and the more a patient will be seen in an office.

Competition is also increasing for the physical therapist. Today, we are seeing more and more alternative forms of health care that border closely on the practice of physical therapy. Many consumers still know little about physical therapy and services which are available from a licensed professional. Changes in the external environment are increasingly forcing each professional to step forward and engage in "turf protection battles."

The Indirect Action Environment

Those factors present in the indirect action environment generally do not have as great of an influence on the health care organization as those in the direct action environment. The indirect action environment is more complex and uncertain. Consequently, the exact effect variables in the indirect action environment have on the organization is uncertain. The factors most influencial in the indirect action environment include: technology, economic variables, sociocultural, and political factors.

Technology

The level of technology plays a significant role in the services a health care organization can offer to the patient. For the hospital, the acquisition of new medical equipment or the addition of a new service can be of tremendous assistance in gaining a competitive edge in a community. The medical technology available today is helping to keep people healthy much longer. Ten years ago, a premature baby weighing one to two pounds at birth stood little chance of surviving. Today, medical science has the ability to save young lives but often at a cost of $100,000 or more. Improvements in technology have made it possible for more than 85,000 kidney, liver, heart, and heart-lung transplants to be performed from 1982 to 1987.[11] The sweeping changes in technology have been more important than anything else in increasing the costs of health care.

Economic Conditions

A hospital's top management must assess the effect changes in economic conditions will have on the organization and its operations. Economic conditions affect the costs of labor, supplies and the ability of the consumer to seek out health care services. If members of top management see the potential for a period of prolonged inflation, they may request all department heads order supplies now in order to hold down costs in the future. They may also seek financing for any proposed construction, especially if interest rates are projected to rise. If, on the other hand, the hospital predicts a decrease in occupancy, they may implement a hiring freeze to maintain costs at acceptable levels.

Economic conditions may strongly influence the private practitioner's attempts to obtain capital for additional equipment or facility expansion. The federal government actively engages in attempts to head off periods of inflation or recession. The government does so through adjustments in taxation, the money supply, and through the interest rates charged by the Federal Reserve Bank. When the Federal Reserve Bank increases its interest rate requirements for loans, these are often followed by the commercial lending institutions. The process of increasing interest rates makes borrowing money more expensive for hospitals and small business professionals such as the private practitioner. When the federal government implements tax cuts it does so to stimulate the production of goods and services as well as to encourage businesses to hire more personnel.

It is important to keep in mind, however, that changes in economic conditions may influence some areas of the economy more than others. The same is true for the physical therapist who ventures into private practice. Those practitioners who locate in regions of the country where the economy is depressed may experience slow growth and encounter higher numbers of uncollectable patient accounts. Those practices located in more affluent regions may notice little or no change in patient volume in the midst of a recession.

Sociocultural Factors

Sociocultural factors such as attitudes, values, and customs influence how an organization and its managers operate. The values important to a hospital or to the owner of a small private practice are reflected in the organization's objectives, goals, and structure. In the American health care system the public has well-established expectations and values about what constitutes quality patient care and ethical practice. Practices such as treating only those patients who can afford to pay will eventually place a stigma on the reputation of the organization. Questions about the quantity of health care a person should receive are also of increasing importance. After all, who should determine how many liver transplants a patient should receive before it is someone else's turn?

Sociocultural factors also affect how the organization makes its services available. With medical costs rising as rapidly as they are, hospitals and physicians are increasingly requesting cash down payments for elective surgery. In some centers, patients who wish to receive non-emergency surgery must cover at least part of the cost of surgery before it is performed.

Sociocultural factors influence how and why hospitals attract patients. Hospitals who are in close proximity of one another are increasingly having to compete for patients in order to remain viable. Instances have been documented where physicians have received thousands of dollars earmarked "thanks for your continued support." Actions such as these serve to drive up the costs of health care for all consumers.

Physical therapists entering into private practice have been unable to escape the difficulties encountered in developing a business. Instances have been reported where physical therapists have been approached and offered lucrative deals to engage in referral for profit. Society recognizes the need for the physical therapist to make a living as long as the services are ethical and cost contained. The independent practitioner rarely can award profits to outside sources and still keep costs and services at reasonable levels.

Political Influence and the Local Community

For many health care organizations the climate in the local community has almost as much bearing on internal operations as does the federal government. As a result of the tremendous political influence which can be exercised at the local level, most hospitals and their administrators cooperate fully with local officials. In many instances, cooperating with local officials may mean nothing more than contributing time or monies to local schools, charities, and fund-raising drives.

The physical therapist must also participate in local community functions if he or she is to be perceived as a viable force in the local economy. The professional must engage in personal selling with members of both the medical and non-medical community. Personal selling is a face-to-face oral interaction between two or more parties for the express purpose of making a positive representation of an individual, organization, product, or service.

Physical therapists are often hesitant about the idea of personal selling. Whether most of us know it or not we engage in personal selling on a daily basis through interactions with medical doctors, patients, and various community contacts. Personal selling is only one small part of making an organization successful.

THE ORGANIZATION, THE ENVIRONMENT, AND CHANGE

As previously noted, there are a number of factors present in the environment which directly and indirectly influence the health care organization and the services offered. Each of these factors will be present throughout the life of the organization and beyond. Understanding and effectively utilizing the systems concept in health care management requires the manager to properly identify and cope with each of these factors. Coping with the environment, and the factors presented, will often require changes be made within the health care organization. Change is a vital part of the organization and a key to its continued survival.

Change in a health care organization usually involves a managerial decision to alter one or more of the internal variables in the organization. Management may consider changes in organizational objectives, structure, technology, or in some of the health care personnel. Decisions of this type can be categorized as either proactive or reactive. A proactive decision is one made in response to something the manager perceives may occur. At the time the decision is made, no problem exists. The change will be made in response to a perceived opportunity in the environment. A reactive change is made in response to a problem. Here, the manager reacts to a problem which has already been identified in the managerial control process.

Systems theory recognizes that no change can be implemented in an organization without its effects being felt elsewhere. As research has shown, a change which focuses on only one aspect or variable in an organization is not as effective as those changes which focus on more than one variable.[12] The following are some of the important areas within an organization that should be considered in a change process.

Objectives

Regardless of the size of the organization, all health care managers should periodically evaluate and, if necessary, change established objectives. Changes should be made in accordance with the demands of the internal and external environment. The need to change will be identified by utilizing the feedback mechanism in the systems concept.

Structure

Changing the structure of an organization refers to changes in the authority/responsibility relationships. Occasionally, membership in the managerial hierarchy will change, necessitating changes in the coordinating and integrating mechanisms within the organization. The impact of the process will be obvious on the organizational chart but may not be as obvious on the personnel involved. Change may be particularly hard on non-managerial personnel because of the requirement of having to establish new reporting relationships.

Technology and Tasks

Changing technology and tasks in an organization refers to changing the way work is processed, patients are scheduled for services, along with the introduction of new forms of medical equipment and technology. As with structural changes, technological changes interrupt reporting relationships and social patterns. The introduction of new technological equipment requires time for employee adjustment. The introduction of change, especially changes in technology, can create a number of uncertainties for the health care employee. Systems theory, and its proper application, forces the manager to recognize some of the uncertainties frequently encountered in technological change.

1) FEAR OF ECONOMIC LOSS. Rapid advances in technology may make some workers, especially those approaching retirement, feel insecure in their jobs. Some employees feel as though their positions will be eliminated, they could be laid off, or terminated before their career is complete. As a health care manager it is important to understand how an employee feels when changes are implemented. The best way to reduce insecurities of this type is to establish effective channels of communication.

2) INCONVENIENCE One of the more common complaints health care managers hear is that of the inconvenience caused by change. Each of us are creatures of habit who mentally and physically resist changes which force the termination of a routine. The health care manager who explains the rationale behind the change helps reduce resistance.

3) FEAR OF UNCERTAINTY. People may resist change because of the feelings of uncertainty it sometimes produces. Feelings of insecurity and uncertainty are easy to understand. The person may not comprehend the intent of the proposed change. Some employees perceive the change as a threat to their inherent need for security. As discussed in Chapter Three, security is considered one of the most basic needs the individual desires to have fulfilled.

STEPS FOR IMPLEMENTING ORGANIZATIONAL CHANGE

Implementing change in a health care organization should follow a few basic steps in order to be successful. All change efforts must recognize the effect they will have on the organization as a system. The manager must identify the interrelationships among variables and approach the change effort with the idea of creating as little confusion as possible. Changes can be introduced by proceeding through the following six steps:

1) RECOGNIZING THE NEED FOR CHANGE. Viewing the health care organization as part of a complex system in a dynamic environment forces the manager to realize changes are needed and that they can be good for the morale of the organization. All changes must have the support of top management in the organization. Without top management support, changes may never be properly introduced or may be introduced to the detriment of the organization. Although most changes are implemented at the top of the organization and directed downward, it is possible to implement changes at the middle or bottom of the organization. As evidenced in Figure 2-5, changes can be introduced at any level but still need top management support in order to be effective.

2) ORGANIZATIONAL REORIENTATION. An organization contemplating change must once again become reacquainted with itself. The concept of organizational reorientation is a top-down and bottom-up

approach. Each manager rediscovers what the organization is all about and where individual departments fit in. This may include redefining the basic mission of the organization as well as redefining its primary objectives and goals.

3) DIAGNOSIS OF THE PROBLEM. Management must gather information concerning the true nature of the problem. Problem definition and analysis often occurs at the top of the organization. Individual department managers may be called upon to contribute ideas and suggestions after the scope of the problem has been identified.

4) COMMITMENT TO CHANGE. Once the problems have been identified, management must develop solutions and determine the degree of resource commitment to the change process. The depth of the change should be determined along with the degree of personnel involvement. Change can be narrow or broad depending on whether it is to be organizational wide or apply to only a few individuals.

5) EXPERIMENTAL CHANGE. Implementing any form of change in a health care organization naturally involves some degree of risk. Those changes which are broad are the most risky. The degree of risk can be reduced by implementing change in one or two departments before implementing it on an organizational-wide basis. This provides the members of management with an opportunity to "work the bugs out." By implementing change on a smaller scale, management can determine if the change is working, how well it is being received, and how it should be readjusted. Experimental change allows the search for negative consequences before organizational implementation.

6) OBTAINING ACCEPTANCE FOR THE CHANGE. The final step for the health care management team is to motivate those subordinates who are responsible for implementing the change. Convincing subordinates to implement a change process must be done through efforts that demonstrate the change is beneficial for both the organization and for the subordinates. To effectively implement a change process the manager must recognize the natural tendency to resist change and take steps to forestall it. According to the "Force Field Theory" of Kurt Lewin, an individual's behavior is the result of an equilibrium between driving and restraining forces.[13] The driving forces are those forces to create change, whereas the restraining forces are those which serve to keep the organization unchanged.

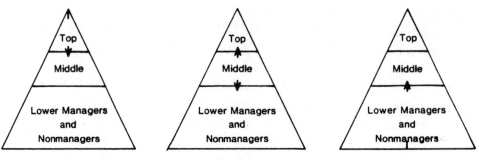

Figure 2-5.

Any behavior we select, or performance level we choose, is a reconciliation between the driving and restraining forces. A proposed model of the force field for the physical therapist is diagrammed in Figure 2-6. This model differs from Lewin's model, in that the physical therapist does not act alone in the care and treatment of patients. There are a number of pressures which drive the therapist toward a behavior. The level of professionalism and the guidance provided by the physician can serve to stimulate the individual to change behavior.

To overcome the obstacles which inhibit change, Schein later developed

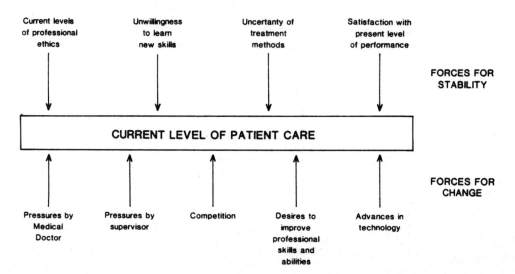

Figure 2-6.

a three-step model that recognizes the need to unfreeze the present behavior pattern, implement the change process, and refreeze the new behavior by reinforcing it.[14] As such, the supervisor of physical therapy would:

1) Unfreeze the old behavior by making it so obvious of the need to change that the individual recognizes it.
2) Changing the behavior involves fostering new ideas, values, and attitudes that will be perceived as necessary for effective performance.
3) Refreezing the behavior by reinforcing it so that it becomes a norm.

All programs of change implemented by the organization and its managers must be directed toward removing the restraining forces and strengthening the driving forces. The idea is that any change that needs to be made will be more effectively accomplished by decreasing the restraining forces rather than by increasing the driving forces. This is especially true in patient care. It is certainly much easier to initially show a patient how to perform an activity correctly rather than spend extended periods of time correcting a bad habit.

OPEN SYSTEMS THINKING AND HEALTH CARE MANAGEMENT

Although health care organizations are clearly open systems, some managers continue to use closed systems thinking when focusing on specific parts of the organization. The physical therapy department is but one subsystem in a larger system. Understanding the systems concept requires an awareness of the interdependency of an organization and its environment. Lacking complete knowledge of the systems concept often leads to the use of "single-cause habit thinking."[15] Single cause thinking is the tendency to look for isolated causes to problems. Few problems have single causes. Upon examination, most problems have multiple causes and reasons. The manager who displays single-cause thinking considers a problem as having a single cause which requires only a single solution.

Systems theory provides the health care manager with a way of looking at the whole picture. General systems theory embraces a major, ongoing attempt to identify how general laws and concepts unify a number of different fields.[16] The manager who utilizes systems theory looks beyond single-cause thinking and tends to be less judgmental. Understanding the interrelatedness and interdependency of an organization with it environment helps the manager diagnosis and identify reasons for effectiveness or ineffectiveness in the health care organization. As one manager explained, "Once a systems point of view prevails, instead of explaining the whole in terms of its parts, parts are explained in terms of the whole."[17]

REFERENCES

1. See, for example, Kenneth E. Boulding, "General Systems Theory—the Skeleton of Science," Management Science, (April 1956), pp. 197–208, and Ludwig Von Bertalanffy, "General Systems Theory—A Critical Review," in Walter Buckley (ed.), Modern Systems Research for the Behavioral Scientist (Chicago: Aldine Publishing Co., 1968).
2. Thomas E. Simonton, "Rep. Stark, Sen. Rockefeller Address Health Issues at APTA Forum," American Physical Therapy Association Progress Report, June 1989, pp. 1–2.
3. Alvar O. Elbing, "On the Applicability of Environmental Models," in J. W. McGuire (ed.), Contemporary Management (Englewood Cliffs, NJ: Prentice-Hall, 1974) p. 283.
4. Gerald D. Bell, "Organizations and the External Environment," in McGuire, op. cit., p. 260.
5. F. W. Emery and E. L. Trist, "The Casual Texture of Organizational Environments," Human Relations, Vol. 18 (1963), pp. 20–26.
6. Steven C. Renn, "The Structure and Financing of the Health Care Delivery System of the 1980's," in Health Care and its Costs, Carl J. Schramm, (ed.), (W. W. Norton, 1987), pp. 29–31.
7. Joan Hamilton, Emily Smith, Susan Garland, "High-Tech Health Care: Who Will Pay?" Business Week, February 6, 1989, pp. 74–78.
8. Renn, "The Structure and Financing of the Health Care Delivery System of the 1980s," p. 45.
9. Stephen W. Brown, Andrew P. Morley Jr., "Marketing Strategies for Physicians," NJ: Medical Economics, 1986, p. 7.
10. Graduate Medical Educational National Advisory Committee Report (1980).
11. Hamilton, "High-Tech Health Care: Who Will Pay?" op., cit. pp. 74–78.
12. Frank Friedlander and L. D. Brown, "Organization Development," Annual Review of Psychology, vol. 25 (1974), p. 314; John P. Campbell and M. D. Dunnette, "Effectiveness of T–Group Experiences in Managerial Training and Development," Psychological Bulletin, vol. 70 (August 1968), pp. 73–104.
13. Kurt Lewin, Field Theory in Social Science: Selected Theoretical Papers (New York: Harper & Brothers, 1951).
14. Kurt Lewin, "Frontiers in Group Dynamics: Concept, Method, and Reality

in Social Science," Human Relations, 1, no. 1. (1947): 5–41. See also Edgar Schein, Organizational Psychology, 3d ed. (Englewood Cliffs, NJ: Prentice-Hall, 1980), pp. 243–247; and Edgar F. Huse and Thomas G. Cummings, Organization Development and Change, 3d ed. (St. Paul, Minn.: West Publishing, 1985), p. 20; William J. McGuire, "Attitudes and Attitude Change," in Gardner Lindzey and Elliot Aronson, eds., Handbook of Social Psychology, 3d ed., vol. 2 (New York: Random House, 1985), chapter 6; and Joel Cooper and Robert T. Croyle, "Attitudes and Attitude Change," Annual Review of Psychology 35 (1984): 395–426.

15. J. Seller, Systems Analysis in Organizational Behavior (Homewood, Ill.: Dorsey Press, 1967), p. 11.

16. C. Churchman, The Systems Approach (New York: Delta Books, Dell Publishing, 1968); F. Kast and J. Rosenzweig, Organization and Management: A Systems Approach (New York: McGraw-Hill, 1974); D. Katz and R. Kahn, The Social Psychology of Organizations (New York: Wiley, 1966); F. Luthans and T. Stewart, "A General Contingency Theory of Management," Academy of Management Review 2 (April 1977): 181–195; and J. Lorsch and J. Morse, Organizations and Their Members: A Contingency Approach (New York: Harper & Row, 1974).

17. R. Ackoff, "A Note on Systems Science," Interfaces 2 (August 1972): 40.

Chapter Three

MOTIVATION: THE FORCE BEHIND EMPLOYEE BEHAVIOR

Health care managers are directly responsible for the quality of patient care provided and the effectiveness of the organization. It has long been recognized that a health care organization's overall performance is directly related to a manager's ability to motivate and lead a group of subordinates. All health care organizations are faced with the fact that vast differences exist in the performance of the individual employees. Some health care professionals perform at high levels, requiring little or no direction and appear to enjoy their job. Others perform at only marginal levels and require constant managerial attention and direction.

There are a number of reasons for the differences in performance. Some of the primary influencing factors include the nature of the job,

58

the behavior of the manager, and the characteristics of the employees. This chapter is concerned with how a health care manager can motivate, influence, direct, and communicate with professionals and non-professionals. The chapter defines motivation and discusses its importance in the health care environment. A health care manager cannot be an effective leader unless employees are motivated to work in a coordinated fashion towards the objectives and goals of the organization.

MOTIVATION TO PROVIDE HEALTH CARE

If the health care manager is to be successful, he or she must have a thorough understanding of the fundamentals of motivation. Understanding motivation is not an easy job because it is an intervening variable; an internal psychological process that the health care manager cannot see. In general, motivation can be defined as a set of processes which sustains an individual's behavior toward the attainment of some objective or goal. In understanding motivation we are interested in what energizes a health care professional's behavior as well as what specific goals they are seeking.

Interestingly enough, those individuals who work hard at providing quality rehabilitative services are often referred to as highly motivated. Those who sit idly for prolonged periods are often critically referred to as unmotivated. The problem with referring to motivation in this manner is that we are essentially measuring only an individual's movement. Motivation is, of course, much more than just the measurement of movement. A physical therapist who sits quietly at a desk and reads a professional journal is someone who is motivated to increase his or her knowledge base. As such, there are two components to motivation. One component is the person's movement, while the other component is the person's motive. Movement, or the lack of it, can easily be seen, whereas a motive can only be inferred. Motives are an individual's needs, desires, or wants which initiate and maintain a given activity. Individual motives are internalized and directed towards a goal.

Many of the factors which assist in motivating the health care professional are difficult to ascertain with certainty. Researchers have developed a number of enlightening theories on the subject of human motivation. Each of these theories differs somewhat in providing recommendations as to what a manager should do to obtain effective performance. It has, however, been the experience of many health care managers that both employees and patients are more encouraged to work towards an objective or goal if they receive occasional encouragement and praise.

Health care managers who make a concerted effort to determine what motivates and satisfies their employees are more likely to develop ways to increase productivity in their department. In the discussion which follows there will be a review of the early theories and more modern views concerning the subject of human motivation. Motivation will be examined regarding its importance to work, behavior and satisfaction. Outwardly, the subject of human motivation may seem quite simple, but it is not. When attempting to study any individual's motivation to perform in the health care environment there must be a careful consideration of the many variables which can influence behavior. Failure of the supervisor to "diagnose" all of the variables affecting an individual's motivation to perform can result in changes being made which are inappropriate and potentially harmful to the health care organization.

WAYS OF LOOKING AT INDIVIDUAL MOTIVATION

There are two broad theory classifications concerning the subject of human motivation. They are the content and process theories of motivation. Content theories focus on "what" arouses, energizes, or starts individual behavior. The basic concept of the content theory is that needs drive a person to behave in a particular manner. A need is an internal quality of someone that arouses specific acts or patterns of behavior. Hunger (the need for food), a steady job (the need for security), or career advancement (the need for promotion) are all examples of such needs.

Process theories focus on the "how" of human motivation. Here, the analysis is of how behavior is energized, directed, maintained, or stopped. Both theories are important to the physical therapist in a supervisory position. Knowing that each person is attracted to a unique set of goals allows the supervisor to plan a motivational process to enhance the individual's chances of achieving their intended outcome.

The Content Theories of Motivation

One of the most widely discussed and simplistic approaches to the study of human motivation are the content theories. Theorists most closely associated with the content theories include Abraham Maslow, Clayton

Alderfer, Fredrick Herzberg, and David McClelland. Each of these theorists attempt to answer the question, "What need is the individual attempting to satisfy?" As such, the content theory attempts to determine what factors within the individual causes them to act or perform in the ways they do.

Probably one of the best known and most popular of the content theories of human motivation is the one developed by Abraham Maslow.[1] As a clinical psychologist, Maslow developed the Hierarchy of Needs, based on the assumption that individuals are motivated to satisfy several different needs. The various needs are arranged in a hierarchy in such a manner that an individual will attempt to satisfy some needs before trying to satisfy others.

Maslow's hierarchial theory defines five need categories. Arranged in order from lowest to highest they are physiological, security, affiliation, esteem, and self-actualization. Maslow's theory assumes that the individual will behave in ways which lead to the satisfaction of their needs. A person will first try to satisfy the most basic needs (physiological) before trying to satisfy the upper level needs (esteem and self-actualization). Once a need has been satisfied, according to Maslow, it ceases to be motivational. Figure 3-1 graphically depicts the Maslow theory.

Description of the Theory

Physiological needs are at the lowest level of the hierarchy. Needs which are considered physiological include food, water and shelter. An individual, according to the theory, will attempt to satisfy those needs before seeking to satisfy higher order needs. In many of the world's most poor and underdeveloped countries, a large segment of the population clings to life solely by attempting to satisfy their physiological needs for food and shelter.

Once physiological needs have been met the individual will then focus on satisfying their needs for security. The individual's need for safety, protection from pain or threat of harm are all considered by Maslow as security needs. In the work place, security needs are expressed most often as a desire for a retirement program, medical insurance, and a working environment which is safe and comfortable. In health care organizations these needs may also be met through guaranteed job security or salary increases that keep up with the cost of inflation.

When physiological and security needs have been satisfied, the indi-

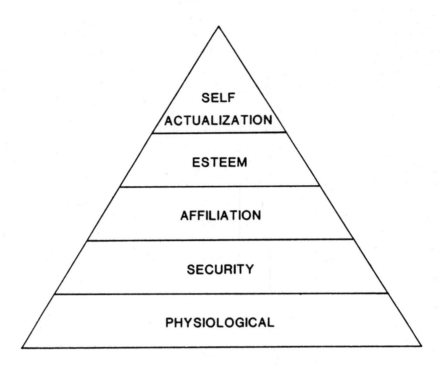

Maslow's Hierarchy of Needs

Figure 3-1.

vidual will become motivated to satisfy affiliation needs. Affiliation is the need for the individual to be social, to have friends, and to be accepted by others. The quality of supervision and professional friendships are critical elements to the individual worker's satisfaction of the need for affiliation.

Esteem is the individual's desire to maintain self-respect and obtain the respect of others. Those individuals who are concerned about their needs for esteem look for opportunities to achieve, obtain increased responsibility, promotion, and recognition of their competence and capabilities. The opportunity to excel at something or solve a problem helps lead to feelings of worth, adequacy, and self-confidence. The individual who does not or cannot satisfy their needs for esteem may increasingly become dissatisfied with their employment situation.

Self-actualization is the need to discover who we are and develop to our fullest potential. The individual desires to maximize the use of his or her skills or abilities. Individuals at the level of self-actualization desire work assignments which challenge their skills, allow them to be creative and provide opportunities for advancement and personal growth.

Individuals at the self-actualization level may experience increased problem-solving ability and have a greater desire for privacy.

Applying Maslow's Theory to Health Care Management

Maslow's theory has been popular among some managers, probably because it is so simple and intuitively appealing.[2] This may be because the practical implications of the theory are many. For example, if an employee is motivated to satisfy physiological needs, he or she will be unlikely to focus on performing the work. The physiological needs must be satisfied by a wage adequate enough to feed, clothe, and shelter the worker's family satisfactorily. A health care manager who strives to motivate employees by appealing to their physiological needs will offer better fringe benefits and improved working conditions. Here, the managerial assumption is that people primarily work for money. They try to motivate employees by offering wage increases to help provide for the physiological needs.

To satisfy the security needs of an employee, the health care manager may focus on emphasizing rules and regulations, job security, and protection against automation. An employee with strong security needs desires a job with safety and long-range protection against layoffs. The same employee may be somewhat less innovative and generally avoids any behavior which causes internal conflict in the organization. The individual who desires security will often do as they are told. It is important that both physiological and security needs be met satisfactorily in a health care organization.

Those people with needs for affiliation value their work as an opportunity to find and establish interpersonal relationships. The individual worker may value social interactions such as the company picnic, the company softball game, or other related activities. A health care manager who recognizes the value of affiliation to an individual employee will encourage loyalty and satisfaction. The health care manager must be careful, however, not to create a situation where a reduction in job performance is caused by employees who place a greater value on their social relationships than on their work.

In the hospital setting, the administrator, or one of the vice-presidents, will fill the role of helping to meet the individual's need for self-esteem. The administrator does this by providing public recognition for outstanding health care services or dedication to the organization. Hospitals frequently recognize and provide rewards for employees with 5, 10, 15 or more years of service to the organization. In other cases, employees will be recognized as having demonstrated unique skills and abilities. The supervisor of a physical therapy department can also enhance an employee's esteem through the recognition of those physical therapists who accept leadership roles in the profession or publish articles in professional journals.

Health care managers who emphasize meeting employee needs for self-actualization frequently involve them in more decision-making opportunities. The supervisor may encourage individual member creativity and suggest the implementation of new or specialized treatment techniques. Those physical therapists who have an interest in self-actualization will seek patient care assignments which are challenging and require the use of their unique skills or abilities.

Support for Maslow's Theory

Maslow's Hierarchy of Needs theory predicts a step-by-step process of motivation in which individual behavior is influenced by a changing set of needs. How much a particular need motivates the individual depends on its position in the need hierarchy and the extent to which it and all lower needs have been satisfied. Maslow did not claim that the hierarchy is rigidly fixed, especially for middle level needs such as affiliation and esteem which may vary from person to person. He does believe that physiological needs are the most basic and self-actualization needs are the least fulfilled. There is, however, insufficient evidence to support the theory that the hierarchy exists for anything but the basic needs.[3] Research does indicate that unless basic needs are satisfied people will not be motivated to satisfy higher level needs.

With research failing to totally support Maslow's theory, Clayton Alderfer proposed a simpler model.[4] Labeled as the ERG theory, Alderfer postulates three needs. They are:

E: Existence
R: Relatedness
G: Growth

As such, the ERG theory is simply a less rigid model than the one developed by Maslow. Existence (physiological and security needs) and relatedness (the need to develop to one's own potential) all follow the same pattern as described by Maslow. In contrast to the Hierarchy of Needs, Alderfer's theory recognizes several needs may exist at the same time and that the basic needs may not be activated in a hierarchial order.

The ERG theory therefore reduces the number of need categories by eliminating the restriction about the order in which needs are activated. It further indicates that one need may be activated regardless of whether or not the other needs are fulfilled. With little evidence indicating that there are five basic needs activated in a hierarchial order, Alderfer's simpler and less restrictive approach may be more applicable to the life of the modern manager than the more confining Maslow theory.

Herzberg's Two-Factor Theory

Fredrick Herzberg developed the two-factor theory of motivation in an attempt to further contribute to an understanding of the relationship between job characteristics and motivation.[5] He and his associates undertook research which investigated the relationship between job satisfaction and worker productivity. Together, they accumulated data on various factors that affected the workers' feelings toward their jobs. This research led to the development of a two-factor theory of motivation identifying hygienic and motivating factors in the work environment.

In Herzberg's initial study, the researchers interviewed over 200 engineers and accountants.[6] The professionals were asked to recall specific events or incidents within the past year that made them feel either good or bad about their jobs. The results of the interviews indicated that in almost all cases those factors which had a stimulating effect on performance were related to job satisfaction. Those factors which had a negative effect on performance were related to job dissatisfaction.

The factors which were associated with positive feelings about the job were labeled motivators. Favorable feelings were related to specific tasks performed, such as doing well at a job and becoming an expert in the field. On the other hand, factors which were unfavorable or related to job dissatisfaction were labeled as hygienics. Based on their findings, a distinction was made between those factors which are hygienic in a job and those which serve as motivators. The factors are depicted in Figure 3-2.

Hygienic and Motivating Factors

Hygiene factors come directly from the organization to which the individual belongs. Herzberg, when using the word *hygiene*, was referring to things the organization can and should do for the workers to prevent them from becoming dissatisfied or unmotivated. Hygienes includes such things as company policies, supervision, working conditions,

HERZBERG'S HYGIENE AND MOTIVATING FACTORS

Hygiene Factors	Motivating Factors
Company Policies and Administration	Achievement
Quality of Technical Supervision	Recognition
Interpersonal Relations	Responsibility
Working Conditions	Advancement
Salary	Challenging Work
Job Security	Possibility of Growth on the Job

Figure 3-2.

salary, and job security. Hygiene factors, by their mere presence, do not lead to job satisfaction. If absent, however, they may lead to dissatisfaction with the job. Herzberg believes that if these factors are not present, workers are likely to become dissatisfied and perform less work.

Motivators are factors which are associated with positive feelings about a job. The motivators are related to the job itself and include such things as achievement, recognition, and advancement. If these factors are present, they will serve to motivate the individual towards superior performance. According to the theory, motivators are crucial factors that serve to stimulate people to do more and better work.

The major difference between motivators and hygienes is that motivators are job centered and related directly to the nature of the job itself. If the job is exciting, presents a challenge, or is rewarding, it will be motivating to the health care professional. Conversely, hygienes are more closely identified with the context in which the work is performed. Herzberg suggests that just because the physical therapy department has some of the most modern and up-to-date equipment does not necessarily mean workers will be more highly motivated to perform than if the department is not well equipped. The workers will simply be less likely to become dissatisfied.

Managerial Application of Herzberg's Theory to the Health Care Environment

Herzberg's theory is an important contribution to modern management. It has made a significant impact on further understanding the effects of job characteristics on individual motivation, satisfaction and job performance. Despite all of its contributions, the theory is not without its critics. Dunnette et al. believe Herzberg's work oversimplifies the nature of job satisfaction.[7] The author states:

Results show that Herzberg's two factor theory is a grossly oversimplified portrayal of the mechanism by which job satisfaction or dissatisfaction comes about. Satisfaction or dissatisfaction can reside in the job context, the job content or both jointly. Moreover, certain job dimensions, notably achievement, responsibility and recognition, are more important for both satisfaction and dissatisfaction than certain job dimensions, notably working conditions, company policies and practices and security.

The primary value to the health care manager is the way the job-related factors are divided into two groups. There are those factors which serve to motivate the employee and those which do not. This is important to recognize, since it implies not everything a manager does will serve to motivate the employee. Hygiene factors such as excellent working conditions may provide little or no motivation. For example, if salary is considered to be low by employee standards, it may become a source of job dissatisfaction and lead to the eventual departure of the employee from the health care organization. Of additional interest is the fact that Herzberg's factors parallel Maslow's concept. Herzberg's motivators relate to the two highest levels (esteem and self-actualization), whereas the maintenance factors relate to the lower level needs, primarily affiliation, security, and the physiological needs (see Figure 3-3).

The subject of job satisfaction is of increasing importance to the health care manager. Some studies report a low to moderate inverse relationship between job satisfaction and employee absences from work. Specifically, the more the person is dissatisfied with the job, the more likely he or she is to be absent from work.[8] Concerning turnover, once again the strength of the relationship between turnover and satisfaction is low to moderate. The lower an individual's level of satisfaction, the more likely the person is to resign and seek other work-related opportunities.[9]

These factors recognize the important role the health care manager plays in providing a motivating work environment. The following are some suggestions for increasing job satisfaction in the health care setting.

1) PROVIDE WORK WHICH IS CHALLENGING. All work-related tasks should be designed so as to be interesting but not overly tiring. The job should provide varied treatment assignments with opportunities to receive feedback concerning performance.

2) GOOD WORKING CONDITIONS. The health care facility should be designed so as to allow employees the opportunity to attain work-related goals. Although "luxury" equipment is not always financially obtainable, the department personnel should have available at least the most essential necessities for proper patient care.

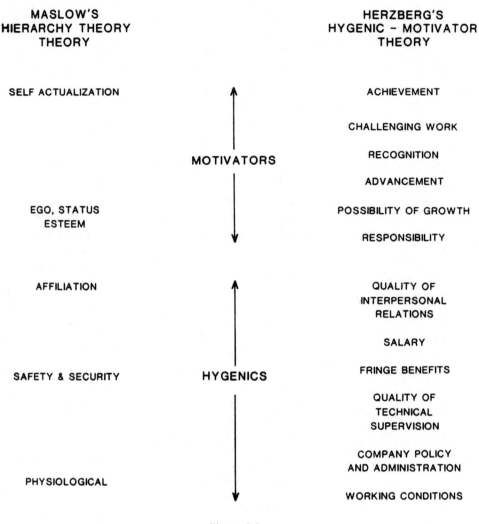

Figure 3-3.

3) RECOGNIZE PERFORMANCE. The health care manager should strive to reward employees for outstanding performance. Providing employee rewards does not always have to be done through bonuses and salary increases. Health care professionals appreciate praise and positive feedback from a supervisor.

4) CREATE A RELAXED CLIMATE. It is the health care manager's responsibility to foster friendly relations between and with co-workers.

5) OUTLINE POLICIES. Clarify all aspects of a job to further enhance an employee's chance of reaching job-related goals.

6) AS SUPERVISOR, DEMONSTRATE YOUR CONCERN. Show a genuine interest in helping employees solve work-related problems. When possible, encourage creativity in problem solving and provide the needed resources to enable the problem to be resolved.

7) PROVIDE A SENSE OF SECURITY. Try to avoid making the employee feel as though his or her job may be at risk.

8) PAY. All health care workers should feel as though they are compensated appropriately and the benefits they are receiving are fair.

9) PROVIDE EMPLOYEES WITH AUTONOMY AND A SENSE OF RESPONSIBILITY. Health care employees often feel they know as much, or more, about their jobs than anyone else. Whenever the department supervisor encounters a problem which affects all employees, solicit the opinions of those most directly involved. Employees will find it gratifying having been consulted by management about important aspects of their jobs.

10) PROVIDE REALISTIC JOB EXPECTATIONS. The health care supervisor should always avoid promising more than can actually be delivered.

Managers should strive to improve the job satisfaction of subordinates. Health care professionals who are high performers are the cornerstones for work groups and organizations. High job satisfaction will generally result in better attendance, reduced turnover and is also of importance psychologically to the individual and to their quality of work life.

McClelland's Theory of Learned Needs

One researcher, taking a somewhat different point of view, believes our needs are as a result of our culture.[10] David McClelland proposed that an organization offers a person the opportunity to satisfy at least three needs. He identified those needs as the need for achievement, the need for affiliation, and the need for power.

According to McClelland, some people have a very strong desire to achieve. They spend a considerable period of time thinking about their jobs and how they can do them better or accomplish important things. They strive to achieve for the sake of achieving rather than for the personal benefits or symbols of success. It has been estimated that approximately 10 percent to 15 percent of the U.S. population possesses a strong need to achieve. Those individuals who have a high need to achieve can often be distinguished from those who have either high needs for affiliation or power. Many of those with high needs to achieve possess the following characteristics:

1) They have a desire to take personal responsibility for a success or failure. Additionally, they like finding a solution to a problem.
2) Most are moderate risk takers. They avoid situations of high or low risk. Specifically, they like goals that are neither too easy nor impossible to achieve.
3) They like to have concrete feedback on their performance.

Individuals with a strong need to achieve often prefer to set their own goals or at least have partial influence in establishing them. They do not like to operate in an environment without goals and are motivated by tasks which provide them with a feeling of competence. Managers with a strong need to achieve often solve problems differently and establish different goals than do managers with high needs for power.[11] Additionally, a high need to achieve seems to be an important factor for those who undertake entrepreneurial activities.[12]

The individual with a high need for affiliation is primarily interested in warm, meaningful and friendly relationships. They particularly prefer an organization where there is social interaction. In contrast to the need for the person to achieve, the manager with a high need for affiliation tends to spend more time communicating with subordinates. As a result of the time spent communicating with subordinates, they are often perceived as good managers who have a genuine interest in the lives of the subordinates.

The person who has a high need for power is someone who is primarily interested in controling situations. The manager with high needs for power can be quite effective when the need is focused outwardly on the organization and not self-aggrandizement. As such, the manager must have a desire to influence others for the good of the organization and not for his or her own personal benefit. The power-motivated manager is more interested in getting things done rather than being liked. The apparently positive connotation or power must, however, be viewed with caution. Evidence suggests that those individuals with high needs for power may suppress the free flow of information if facts contradict their preferred course of action.[13] When important information is suppressed, it can have a profound influence on decision making and group productivity.

The Process Theories of Motivation

The previous section examined four content theories of human motivation. Each of these theories had one thing in common; that is, each was concerned with what is within the individual or the environment that stimulates or sustains behavior. They looked for specific needs that motivate people and result in their subsequent behavior.

The process theories of human motivation are primarily concerned with explaining how behavior is initiated, directed, sustained, and halted. Each of the content theories, while identifying the key work-related elements that energize behavior, provide little information as to why an individual chooses a particular behavior to satisfy a need. The process theory of motivation recognizes the individual is motivated to behave based on the rewards associated with a given behavior. The individual has either seen a specific behavior rewarded or has been told that a certain behavior will be rewarded.

There are three process models of motivation the health care manager should become familiar with. The first and probably the most popular is the expectancy theory. A second popular theory is that of operant conditioning, sometimes referred to as either behavior modification or reinforcement theory. A third theory, the equity theory, asserts that people are motivated to maintain fair relationships with others and will attempt to rectify unfair relationships by making them fair. Each of these theories is discussed below.

The Expectancy Theory

The expectancy theory, developed by Victor Vroom, defines motivation as a process governing choices among alternative forms of voluntary activity.[14] According to Vroom, most behaviors are under the voluntary control of the person. The choice of behavior is the one which can lead to the desired rewards. As such, the individual will evaluate among various strategies of behavior and subsequently choose a behavior that they believe will lead to rewards or work-related outcomes.

Victor Vroom believes people are motivated towards work if they (a) expect that increased effort will lead to a reward and (b) value the rewards that occur as a result of their efforts. From a health care manager's point of view individual motivation would be as follows:

The Individual's Motivation to Perform	=	Chances that Effort will Result in Rewards	×	Value of Rewards to the individual

To understand the expectancy theory involves a familiarity with three main variables: expectancy, valence, and motivation. The primary functions of each of these variables can be explained by the fact that employees determine in advance what their behavior may accomplish and place a value on alternative possible accomplishments or outcomes. The three variables are defined as follows:

1) Expectancy is what the individual anticipates will occur as a result of a given behavior. An individual's expectancy is the perception of probability that a specific result will follow a specific act. The range is similar to that found in statistical probability, namely, 0 to $+1$. The value for certainty would approach $+1$, whereas the value for conditions of uncertainty would be closer to zero. For example, physical therapist Joan Smith has decided that she would like to pursue a career in health care management. She has been carefully considering three options which could potentially lead to her fulfilling that goal. Based on her evaluation she has assigned probabilities to the following methods by which to gain entrance to a management position.

1) Return to school and obtain a master's degree in business administration. 0.85
2) Return to school and obtain a master's degree in physical therapy. 0.75
3) Seek an entry level management position and work to gain experience in the field. 0.50

The first choice, referring to school and obtaining a master's degree, was assigned the highest probability. Joan believes that a business degree will be of assistance in her career if she decides to leave health care administration and enter the private practice setting. The other alternatives, returning to school for a master's degree in physical therapy or seeking out an entry level management position, are considered important by Joan but are not considered as significant as the business degree.

When evaluating and establishing probabilities it is important to recognize that expectancy is highly influenced by what has occurred in the past. The individual may assign his or her probabilities based on the observations of others and the rewards they have received. In the hypothetical Joan Smith case, her assignment of probabilities was highly influenced by two close friends who had rapidly advanced into health care management after obtaining master's degrees in health services management and business administration.

2) Valence is the strength of an individual's preference for an expected outcome. The individual's preference for a particular outcome may range on a scale from +1 to −1. In the Joan Smith example, the therapist may have a strong and positive preference to either obtaining a master's degree in business administration or in physical therapy. She may, at this time, have a negative interest in seeking a managerial position. The following assigns valences to each of the choices (Figure 3-4).

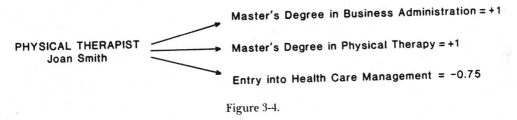

PHYSICAL THERAPIST
Joan Smith

Master's Degree in Business Administration = +1

Master's Degree in Physical Therapy = +1

Entry into Health Care Management = −0.75

Figure 3-4.

3) Motivational force, the foundation of the expectancy theory, is the sum of both expectancy and valence. The motivational force of the individual will be high or low based on the selected values of expectancy and valence. The computation of the motivational force requires simple multiplication. The potential career choices of Joan Smith can be used to illustrate how a final decision can be reached. In reaching her final decision, Joan combines the previous calculations into one number. The number represents the motivation force behind each of the three career alternatives:

	Expectancy	×	Valence	=	Motivational Force
Master's Degree in B.A.	0.85		+1		0.85
Master's Degree in P.T.	0.75		+1		0.75
Management Position	0.50		−0.75		−0.38

Based on the above calculations, returning to school to obtain a master's degree in business administration provides the greatest motivational force. Joan is most likely to return to school and work towards that degree. The other positive motivational force, obtaining a master's degree in physical therapy, is also attractive but not to the same level as the business degree. From the previous calculations, Joan obviously considers seeking an entry level management job as very undesirable.

The Expectancy Theory in Health Care

The expectancy theory stresses that an individual will select a behavior that will result in obtaining valuable rewards. Obviously, it is impossible for the health care manager to determine the motivational force behind each employee in every situation. It is, therefore, the health care manager's job to determine how to most effectively increase the motivation of all employees so the current level of health care can be enhanced. To do so, health care managers should consider the following:

1) IDENTIFY THE EXPECTED LEVELS OF PERFORMANCE. The manager must clearly identify what are considered good, average, and poor levels of performance. The employee should fully understand what constitutes the appropriate behavior, what is to be done, and how rewards are to be provided. Subordinates can only develop a motivational force after the manager has outlined what is expected and how it should be done.

2) DO NOT SET GOALS TOO HIGH. The health care manager must be careful to establish realistic goals for each employee. An employee should have the necessary skills, abilities and resources to complete an assigned task. Goals which are too high and cannot be attained may become a source of employee frustration.

3) ASCERTAIN THE VALUED REWARDS. Every employee has a different set of values and as such recognizes some rewards as more important than others. In order to motivate an employee, the health care manager needs to know what are the valued rewards. Some employees value praise and recognition while others work hard to gain increases in pay or promotions.

The expectancy theory is not without its share of critics.[15] One of the major criticisms of the theory is that it is too complex. The theory is, however, valuable if for no other reason than the fact it emphasizes that motivation involves both arousal and a behavioral choice.

Operant Conditioning

The second process theory of motivation is one which emphasizes the application of rewards by the health care manager. Operant conditioning, also commonly referred to as positive reinforcement or behavior modification, has its foundations in the work of B.F. Skinner.[16] The theory suggests that a person's motivation is a function of its rewards. Behavior which is followed by satisfying consequences tends to be repeated, whereas behavior followed by unsatisfying consequences tends not to be repeated.[17]

According to the theory, people behave the way they do as a result of previous experiences. They have learned that some behaviors result in pleasant outcomes while other behaviors are associated with unpleasant outcomes. In almost all cases, people are more likely to desire pleasant rather than unpleasant outcomes.

The theory of operant conditioning is in sharp contrast to the need and expectancy theories of motivation. Instead of relying on inferences about an individual's internal state, as the Maslow and Herzberg theories do, this theory emphasizes the tendency for the individual to repeat behavior. That is, behavior will be repeated depending on the consequences of past behavior.

The theory of operant conditioning introduces an important concept in the process of motivation. The concept is that of learning. That is, motivated behavior is learned behavior. Through experience, the physical therapist learns the proper methods by which to provide rehabilitative services. In a similar manner, the supervisor learns how to manage a group of health care professionals. Managers can learn to be good managers or poor managers in the same way subordinates learn over time what is considered acceptable and unacceptable performance. The theory can be illustrated as shown in Figure 3-5.

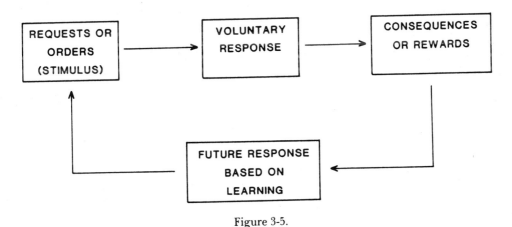

Figure 3-5.

The administration of consequences or rewards is the crucial element by which the person learns acceptable or motivational behavior. In order to determine acceptable behavior the theory focuses on objective and measurable behavior. Adherence to a budget or to a time schedule are examples of objective measures. It is important to recognize that the rewards provided reinforce acceptable levels of behavior and shape the future performance of the individual.

Types of Reinforcement

Undoubtedly, the most distinguishing characteristic differentiating operant conditioning from the other theories of human motivation as presented by Maslow, Herzberg and Vroom is the focus on objective and measurable behavior. There are four types of reinforcement which the health care manager can use to modify or motivate individual behavior. The objective of reinforcement is to change a person's behavior pattern so as to direct them towards more suitable goals. The four types of reinforcement are: positive reinforcement, punishment, extinction and avoidance (see Figure 3-6).

METHODS OF REINFORCEMENT

TYPE OF REINFORCEMENT	STIMULUS	RESPONSE	CONSEQUENCE
Positive Reinforcement	Bonuses result from hard work	Hardwork	Salary increase
Punishment	Repeated absences will not be tolerated	Repeated absences	Employee dismissal
Extinction	Use of improper language by staff member	Manager ignores language	Language improves
Avoidance	Repremands for repeated tardiness	Punctual	No repremand

Figure 3-6.

1) POSITIVE REINFORCEMENT. Any outcome which is pleasant and encourages the individual to repeat a given behavior is called positive reinforcement. Positive reinforcement will be used to increase the likelihood that an individual's behavior will be repeated. Examples of positive reinforcement which can be used by managers in the health care environment include praise, money, and promotions.

2) PUNISHMENT. The managerial use of punishment tells a subordinate what exactly should not be done. The application of negative consequences decreases the likelihood that an undesired behavior will be repeated. The health care manager who utilizes punishment may, for example, provide harsh criticism for an action or limit an individual employee's privileges. Punishment may result in some negative consequences, since it only tells the employee what should not be done rather than what is expected. As a result of the punishment, the employee may develop a negative attitude toward the activity which lead to the punishment, or toward the supervisor and health care organization.

3) EXTINCTION. The health care manager who utilizes extinction ignores the undesired employee behavior. Extinction is, as such, the absence of reinforcement following an unwanted behavior. Physical therapists frequently employ the use of extinction on patients who demonstrate disruptive or improper behavior. Rather than confront the patient, the physical therapist attempts to ignore the behavior and continue the rehabilitative session. The therapist or health care supervisor utilizes this approach with the idea in mind that behavior which is ignored will eventually disappear or become "extinct."

4) AVOIDANCE. The application of avoidance, like positive reinforcement, is used by health care managers to strengthen the reoccurrence of desired behavior. The employee performs the desired behavior to avoid being punished. The distinction between avoidance and positive reinforcement should be clearly made. With positive reinforcement, the employee is rewarded for the desired behavior, whereas with avoidance the employee performs so as to avoid being punished.

The Schedules of Reinforcement

For any method of reinforcement to be effective there must be a careful consideration concerning the element of time. The closer the reinforcement is to the actual behavior, the greater the impact it will have on the employee. There are two broad classifications which consider the element of time. There are those methods of reinforcement which are done on a continuous basis and those which are done on an intermittent schedule.

Reinforcing behavior on a continuous basis is virtually impossible in the health care setting. A manager cannot possibly supervise every activity performed in a department and provide feedback concerning its performance. For reasons of practicality, the health care manager must rely on the intermittent schedule of reinforcement.

The intermittent reinforcement of behavior can be performed in a number of different ways. Reinforcing behavior after a specific period of time is called the *interval schedule.* A reinforcement which is delivered after a certain number of responses is referred to as the *ratio schedule of reinforcement.* The managerial use of the ratio schedule requires a certain number of acceptable employee behaviors before delivering the reinforcement.

The interval schedule of reinforcement can be subdivided into either a fixed or variable format. Managerial use of the fixed-interval schedule requires a specific period of time to pass before reinforcement is applied. The fixed-interval schedule is evidenced when the employee receives a bimonthly paycheck (reinforcement). The variable-interval schedule requires the manager to use a time interval that varies around an average number. The behavior may, for example, be reinforced after the second, sixth, tenth and eighteenth day. The behavior is reinforced on an average of every nine days.

The fixed ratio of reinforcement schedule involves reinforcing a behavior after a fixed number of acceptable behaviors have occurred. The manager may, for example, reinforce behavior after every seventh correct performance. Managerial use of the variable-ratio schedule also requires a certain number of responses before the reinforcement is delivered. The number will, however, vary around an average. Reinforcement may occur after the fifth, ninth, twentieth, twenty-fourth, and thirtieth behavior, or on average after twenty-two occurrences.

Research has shown that the variable-ratio schedule is the most beneficial to sustaining motivated behavior.[18] The reason the variable-ratio schedule is the most effective is because the reinforcement is closely tied to the behavior of the individual and is given closer in time to the actual behavior.

These findings do have a significant impact on the job of the health care manager. In most organizations the employee performance review and salary adjustments are conducted on either a semi-annual or annual basis. Those managers who withhold positive or negative feedback until the performance evaluation accomplish little in changing employee behavior. In order to implement any change in behavior the manager must provide feedback on employee performance throughout the entire employment period, not just once or twice a year.

To fully benefit from the use of operant conditioning, the health care manager may wish to implement some of the following:

1) OUTLINE WHAT IT TAKES FOR THE EMPLOYEE TO RECEIVE POSITIVE REINFORCEMENT. Let each employee know what performance is expected and the rewards that are available. When rewards are outlined, the employees can plan and organize their work and their behavior.

2) REWARD THE BEHAVIOR. For a schedule of reinforcement to be effective it is imperative that the employee be rewarded for the appropriate behavior. In some cases you may need to do nothing more than openly express "a job well done." Unless behavior is at least partially rewarded there is likely to be a decrease in the employee's motivation to perform.

3) VARY THE REWARDS. If every employees' behavior is rewarded the same, essentially ignoring those individuals who perform at above average levels, morale and motivation are likely to suffer. Organizations often give equal wage increases, such as 5 percent, across the board. This fails to recognize those employees who have demonstrated superior performance. The manager must provide rewards which clearly distinguish between the high and low performers.

4) ALWAYS TELL THE EMPLOYEE, IN A RESPECTABLE MANNER, WHAT THEY ARE DOING WRONG. One of the most difficult responsibilities of the health care manager is to criticize an employee's behavior or their performance. If, however, they are expected to improve their performance they need to know where defects in performance lie. All criticisms of employee performance should be done in private. A public reprimand will humiliate the employee and increase resentment towards the manager.

The theory of operant conditioning provides positive implications for the health care managers. Critics are quick to point out, however, that the theory manipulates and controls the individual and their behavior rather than reinforcing it.[19] Properly applied, the theory does not need to exploit the individual. The benefit of the theory is derived from its intent. If the manager utilizes the theory to help the individual worker achieve objectives and goals and thereby greater rewards, the worker will indeed benefit from its managerial application.

The Equity Theory: Social Comparison and Motivation

Throughout our working career each of us will occassionally evaluate what we have compared to what others have. J.S. Adam's equity theory asserts that people are motivated to maintain fair relationships with each other and will attempt to rectify unfair relationships by making them fair.[20] One of the methods for determining fairness in our relationships with others is by social comparison.[21] As such, we get to know ourselves better by comparing ourselves to others. The theory applied to the work environment says that workers make comparisons of one another with respect to outcomes received for inputs into their jobs.

The individual's inputs include how hard the person works at their job, how long he or she has been working, as well as the individual's training, experience, and background. Outcomes include the pay, benefits, and rewards the person receives. The two are compared in the form of a ratio (O/I). The fairness of the ratio is judged not only by the ratio of a person's inputs to outputs, but also as to how the ratio compares to the inputs and outputs of others.

There exists inequity when the two ratios are not equal. For example, if physical therapist "A" believes she has more experience than physical therapist "B," then "A" may believe "B" is overpaid relative to "A." Additionally, since "A" believes she is more experienced than "B," she may feel as though she deserves a raise to be above the salary of "B." As demonstrated below, physical therapist "B" has the more favorable ratio.

$$\frac{\text{P.T. "A" (O)}}{\text{P.T. "A" (I)}} < \frac{\text{P.T. "B" (O)}}{\text{P.T. "B" (I)}}$$

As a result of the perceived inequity, physical therapist "A" will be motivated to reduce the feelings of inequity. Among the actions to be taken, according to Adams, is to reduce the inequity by changing the level of outputs. In other words, physical therapist "A" may begin to work harder or pursue other methods to reduce the inequity. In most cases, the individual will not leave the employment situation unless the inequity is very high and there is no easy way to reduce it.

For the health care manager the theory does have some significance. Analyzing why some employees do not get along with one another may uncover feelings of inequity. Once the feelings have been uncovered and thoroughly discussed, the supervisor can then take the appropriate steps to reduce the source of inequity.

MOTIVATION AND THE SUPERVISOR OF PHYSICAL THERAPY

As this chapter has reported, there are a number of theories concerning the subject of human motivation and behavior in the work place. Each of these theories provides a somewhat different perspective of how best to motivate employees. No one theory provides everything the health care manager needs in order to motivate the professional and non-professional employee. How then does the manager best utilize these theories in the health care environment?

In order to ensure the proper use of any theory concerning the subject of human behavior and motivation, the manager must become a well-versed diagnostician. The manager must realize that any problem within a health care organization may be as a result of a complex interaction of individual needs, behaviorial choices, ability, the rewards offered, and the satisfaction provided by the job. Money, for example, may be a primary motivating tool for one person, while another may be more motivated by the nature of the job.

Applying theory to the health care environment also requires the manager to recognize that individual motivation is a learning process. Every employee comes to an organization with certain preconceived ideas about what their performance should be and how they should behave. The health care manager should not expect results overnight. Attempting to change behavior or motivate employees can be a slow and delicate process. Richard Steers and Lyman Porter suggest the following:[22]

1) Managers must take an active role in managing motivational processes at work. Motivating subordinates is a conscious, intentional behavior, not something that just happens.

2) Managers must understand their own strengths and limitations and have a clear idea of their own desires and wants before attempting to change those of others.

3) Managers should be sensitive to differences in employees. As such, the manager should recognize that different employees have different preferences for rewards. The manager who is aware of the variations in needs, abilities, and traits can more efficiently utilize subordinate talents.

4) Rewards should be based on performance. When employees are rewarded, their expectations generally increase. This should lead to a greater effort toward goal attainment.

5) An employee's job should offer challenge, diversity, and opportuni-

ties for satisfaction. The manager should indicate what level of performance is expected and strive to increase the individual's role clarity.

6) Management should evaluate the quality of the work environment. An organization should be designed so as to limit the number of barriers to task accomplishment.

7) Managers need to continually assess worker attitudes. By staying close to employees, management can identify potential trouble spots. Knowing the personality of each employee allows the manager to act based on objective information rather than on uncertainty.

8) Employee cooperation and support are important to improving organizational output. Employees should have input as to what happens in the organization. They are, after all, also stakeholders in the organization.

REFERENCES

1. A. H. Maslow, Motivation and Personality (New York: Harper & Row, 1954).
2. F. Tuzzolino, & B. R. Armandi, "A Need-Hierarchy Framework for Assessing Corporate Social Responsibility," Academy of Management Review, 1981, 6, 21–28.
3. For Reviews of the literature, see: M. Wahba & L. Bridwell, Maslow Reconsidered: "A Review of Research on the Need Hierarchy Theory." Organizational Behavior and Human Performance, 15, 1976, 212–240; and J. Miner, Theories of Organizational Behavior (Hinsdale, IL: Dryden Press, 1980), pp. 18–43.
4. C. P. Alderfer, Existence, Relatedness, and Growth: Human Needs in Organizational Settings (New York: Free Press, 1972).
5. F. Herzberg, B. Mausner & B. Synderman, The Motivation to Work (New York: John Wiley & Sons, 1959).
6. Ibid.
7. M. Dunnette, J. Campbell, & M. Hakel, "Factors Contributing to Job Dissatisfaction in Six Occupational Groups," Organizational Behavior and Human Performance, May 1967, p. 147.
8. L. W. Porter, & R. M. Steers, "Organizational Work, and Personal Factors in Employee Turnover and Absenteeism," Psychological Bulletin, 1973, 80, 151–176.
9. C. E. Michaels & P. E. Spector, "Causes of Employee Turnover: A Test of the Mobley, Griffeth, Hand, and Meglino Model," Journal of Applied Psychology, 1982, 67, 53–59.
10. David C. McClelland, "Business Drive and National Achievement," Harvard Business Review, July–August 1962, pp. 99–112.

11. J. Hall, "To Achieve or Not: The Manager's Choice," California Management Review 18 (1976): pp. 5–8.

12. D. C. McClelland and D. H. Burnham, "Power Is The Great Motivation," Harvard Business Review, 54 (1976): pp. 100–110.

13. E. M. Fodor & T. Smith, "The Power Motive as an Influence on Group Decision Making," Journal of Personality and Social Psychology, 1982, 42, pp. 178–185.

14. V. H. Vroom, Work and Motivation (New York: John Wiley & Sons, 1964).

15. See F. Schmidt, "Implication of a Measurement Problem for Expectancy Theory Research," Organizational Behavior and Human Performance (April 1973): pp. 243–251; and J. M. Feldman, H. J. Reitz, and R. J. Hilterman, "Alternatives to Optimization in Expectancy Theory," Journal of Applied Psychology (December 1976): pp. 712–720.

16. See B.F. Skinner, Contingencies of Reinforcement (New York: Appleton-Century-Crofts, 1969); and R. M. Tarpy, Basic Principles of Learning (Glenview, IL: Scott, Foresman, 1974).

17. Edward L. Thorndike, Human Learning (New York: Century, 1931).

18. F. Luthans and R. Kreitner, Organizational Behavior Modifications (Glenview, IL: Scott, Foresman, 1975).

19. W. C. Hamner, "Reinforcement Theory and Contingency Management in Organizational Settings," in Organizational Behavior and Management: A Contingency Approach, H. L. Tosi and W. C. Hamner, eds. (Chicago, IL: St. Clair, 1974), pp. 104–108.

20. J. S. Adams, "Inequity in Social Exchange," in L. Berkowitz (Ed.), Advances in Experimental Social Psychology (Vol. 2), New York: Academic Press, 1965.

21. P. S. Goodman, "An Examination of Referents Used in the Evaluation of Pay," Organizational Behavior and Human Performance, 1974, 12, pp. 170–195.

22. Richard M. Steers & Lyman W. Porter, Motivation and Work Behavior, 3rd ed. (New York: McGraw-Hill, 1983), pp. 642–643.

Chapter Four

THE MANAGERIAL ROLE OF
LEADERSHIP IN HEALTH CARE

THE NATURE OF LEADERSHIP
POWER AND LEADERSHIP
GUIDELINES FOR USING POWER IN HEALTH CARE
THEORY X AND THEORY Y: ASSUMPTIONS HELD BY MANAGERS
APPROACHES TO STUDYING LEADERSHIP
   The Trait Approach
   Behavioral Theory
      Supportive Leadership
      Participative Leadership
      Instrumental Leadership
   Contingency/Situational Approaches
      The Tannenbaum and Schmidt Model
      Fiedler's Contingency Theory
      Situational Leadership and The Life Cycle Theory
HEALTH CARE LEADERSHIP:
SOME THOUGHTS ON MANAGERIAL ACTION

Think back to the many organizations which you have belonged to in your lifetime. These may include groups and organizations which were formalized for a specific purpose or for an informal activity. Is there any one thing that each of these organizations or groups had in common? Chances are there is. In almost every case there was one person who was considered "in charge." In each organization whether it be formal or informal in nature, there is usually one person who could influence, direct, or shape the course of events more than anyone else. These key individuals are usually described as leaders.

Effective managerial leadership ability is one of the most important skills a health care manager can possess. Leadership helps bond together the organization and its plans. Leadership is a skill that makes things happen. It is a quality that is respected and admired but is also very elusive to many people.

Leaders play a crucial role in the functioning of all organizations, especially those in health care. Leadership in health care is defined as the exercise of a special influence by one member of the health care organization over others in the same organization. In most health care organizations the leader is appointed to a position of authority. In some situations, however, the leader may be selected by members of the health care organization or emerges in some informal fashion.

Regardless of how an individual becomes a leader it is clear they play a key role in the functioning of the individual group or the organization they are leading. The leader influences attitudes and expectations which serves to encourage or discourage performance. This same ability to influence can also serve to secure or alienate employee commitment to the organization. The general acceptance of the importance of leadership has created a desire in many health care professionals to know more about it. This chapter investigates some of the major theories of leadership and discusses their application in health care.

THE NATURE OF LEADERSHIP

It has long been recognized that an organization's overall performance is related to the quality and effectiveness of the leader. Leaders have, of course, been around for thousands of years. Through the course of time many theories have been developed which have attempted to explain why some individuals are good leaders while others are not. Even though leadership has been extensively studied, scholars have not arrived at a universally agreed upon definition. Some of the more popular definitions of leadership include:

- Leadership is the person who creates the most effective change in group performance.[1]
- Leadership is effective influence.[2]
- Leadership is the exercise of authority and the making of decisions.[3]
- Leadership is the process of influencing group activities toward goal setting and goal achievement.[4]

Each of these definitions points to a common theme; that is, leadership involves influencing other people. The concept of influencing other people is especially true in health care where some individuals are able to influence others by way of their position in the organization, professional abilities, or their educational background. Leadership, as such, must always involve other individuals or groups where there has been a combination of talents and efforts to perform a specific task. Regardless of the situation, the ability or capacity of the individual to influence others must be granted by those health care professionals who are being led. True leadership always involves the willingness of others to recognize an individual as a leader and follow their prescribed directives.

It is also important to recognize that leadership is not the same as management. Leadership is an activity that consists of influencing the behavior of others, both individually and as a group. Management does involve leadership, but it also includes the managerial functions of planning, organizing, staffing, and controlling. The physical therapist who is a manager may not necessarily be a leader. Likewise, the physical therapist who is a recognized leader may not be a manager. A manager occupies a position of authority which has been granted by the administration of the organization. A leader is determined not just by the position of authority but also by those who are being led.

POWER AND LEADERSHIP

Within all health care organizations, managers use power to achieve an interpersonal influence through which leadership is ultimately exercised. Power is an essential leadership resource that, when successfully activated, makes things happen. Unfortunately, the word *power* often carries with it a negative connotation that has undertones of manipulation. In the health care environment it is not uncommon for the professional to be uneasy with the term, especially since it has become recognized as authoritarian behavior. Authoritarian behavior is often expressed in terms of dominance/submission where one person is regarded as a pawn to be used whenever the need arises. This, however, need not be the case. Power can be viewed in a positive way and be of great value to the health care manager.

In the practice of management, power is a term used to describe someone who is successful in getting things done while at the same time rallying support from the people within the work unit. A health care manager who gets things done is one who:

- Provides good jobs for subordinates.
- Obtains above average salary increases for those members of the department.

- Obtains approval for expenditures which extend beyond the budget.
- Has access to the top members of management.
- Can provide information or input concerning decisions and policy-making.

One researcher has suggested that the need for power is essential for executive success.[5] In this instance the individual's need for power is not a need to control for personal satisfaction but rather a desire to influence and control others for the benefit of the organization. Viewing power in a positive way helps to make the study and application of the term much easier.

In an organization there are five sources or bases of power.[6] Each of the five may appear at any level within the organization. They are:

REWARD POWER. In the health care environment, as well as in business or industry, a manager who can provide bonuses, promotions, or increases in pay has reward power. Health care employees will comply with the wishes of the supervisor to the extent to which they believe the supervisor can provide rewards. The rewards may be monetary and non-monetary, such as a salary increase or providing a compliment for a job well done.

COERCIVE POWER. This is the opposite of reward power and involves the manager's ability to punish. Punishment may include a demotion, the docking of pay, or the dismissal of an employee who repeatedly fails to comply with a supervisory request. The health care manager who utilizes coercive power must proceed with caution. Subordinates who are punished may become resentful or hostile. The use of coercive power may also adversly affect an employee's motivation to perform.

REFERENT POWER. This form of power is based on the follower's identification with the leader. The leader is admired because of one or more personal traits and, as a result, can more easily influence followers. The leader also leaves the impression with subordinates that he or she is competent in the performance of the job and is interested in their individual welfare.

LEGITIMATE POWER. This type of power is based upon the individual's position in the hierarchy of the organization. For example, the director of physical therapy possesses more power than the assistant director of physical therapy. Every managerial position in a health care organization possesses legitimate power.

EXPERT POWER. This form of power is held by those individuals who possess some technical expertise, skill, or knowledge that gains them the respect and compliance of subordinates. Individuals who have demonstrated the ability to analyze and control group tasks are often seen as knowledgeable and competent in their jobs. The surgeon, for example, is recognized as an expert because of the advanced training required for professional standing as well as a unique ability to guide other professionals toward desired medical results. Increasingly, the physical therapist is gaining recognition as an expert by assuming greater roles in health care planning, patient treatment, and education.

The degree and scope of a manager's expert and referent power is closely associated with the nature of the leader and with the leader's traits, beliefs, and skills. Some managers possess outward qualities, such as an ability to appear confident in performing a task, while others have the ability to express themselves well.

Coercive, reward, and legitimate power are based upon an individual's position within the organization. The chief executive officer is obviously at a higher managerial level than the director of physical therapy. Consequently, the chief executive officer will possess more coercive, reward, and legitimate power than the director of physical therapy.

GUIDELINES FOR USING POWER IN HEALTH CARE

From the previous discussion, it is clear that a leader's ability to influence is a function of both individual and organizational factors. To properly use power in a health care organization, the manager should consider the following:

1) BE THE BOSS. Once you have been placed in a position of authority, respond in a professional manner. Keep actions consistent with the expectations of others. Inconsistent behavior weakens your power base.
2) GO BEYOND WHAT IS EXPECTED. Whenever possible, go beyond whatever it is that the subordinate expects. Doing favors for others enhances your power position and gains respect from subordinates.
3) BE YOURSELF. Allow other members of the department and organization to get to know you. If the manager is recognized as a good role model, he or she is more likely to command the respect of subordinates.
4) BE AN EXPERT. Allow others to recognize your superiority as a

professional and as a manager. Visable achievements are the foundation on which a reputation is built.

5) OBTAIN THINGS FOR OTHERS. One of the best ways to develop managerial power is to obtain scarce resources for subordinates which they would otherwise be unable to obtain for themselves.

6) DEVELOP CREDIBILITY. If you say something can be done, then be willing to take the responsibility for seeing that it is accomplished.

7) EXERCISE SELF-CONTROL. Avoid egotistical displays of power. Above all, the manager should strive to act with sensitivity and discretion.

When placed in a position which provides an opportunity to exercise power, the physical therapist must proceed with caution. Seldom do people like having power forced upon them. Powerful people often get more things done because someone else enjoys doing an activity rather than because they need to be rewarded. The director of physical therapy must be sensitive to how influence attempts are received. It is not always a matter of getting the job done as much as it is how the manager goes about getting the job done.

THEORY X AND THEORY Y: ASSUMPTIONS HELD BY MANAGERS

All managers have ideas concerning the way in which they would like to see their subordinates behave in the performance of their jobs. Theory X and Theory Y are two separate and distinct sets of assumptions that managers can make about human nature. They are not scientific theories of leadership and supervision but rather working theories or assumptions about subordinates and managers. Douglas McGregor, the originator of the research, believes managers have one of these two philosophies regarding why employees work and how they can best be motivated.[7]

A manager who embraces Theory X asserts that workers must be motivated by pressure applied by management. The manager has the view of the worker as being lazy, lacking ambition, disliking responsibility and as someone who prefers to be led. The manager must, therefore, elicit desired behavior through the offering of financial incentives and managerial control. If tight controls are ineffective, it may become necessary to use coercion and threats of punishment in order to obtain the desired work behavior.

In contrast, Theory Y assumes that people will become self-motivated to achieve organizational goals as a natural consequence of their striving for personal growth and development. A Theory Y manager maintains a more trusting and open relationship with an employee. The alternative assumption is made that the average employee does like work and therefore considers work as natural as either play or rest. The worker is considered a self-directed adult who is committed to organizational objectives and goals. A Theory Y manager sees an employee as capable of being self-motivated and that threats of punishment or coercion are not the only way to direct employee effort toward performance.

What type is most often seen in the health care environment: Theory X or Theory Y? Think back to one of the more recent health care managers you have had the opportunity to work with. Was this person an individual who attempted to control every aspect of patient care and departmental policy? Or, in contrast, was the supervisor someone who was more expressive with individual employee freedom while encouraging a warm and friendly working environment?

It is indeed rare to find a health care manager who is entirely Theory X. Most are to some degree a "soft Theory X." While many health care managers agree that both professional and non-professional employees work hard at patient treatment tasks, there are those times when they do not. Managers often feel employees take advantage of the situation by sustaining self-direction and effort for only short periods of time. There are, however, many physical therapy departments throughout the United States where the Theory Y concept is an accurate description of managerial assumptions about professional and non-professional employees.

APPROACHES TO STUDYING LEADERSHIP

The subject of leadership has been the object of considerable study, research, and debate. Every health care organization needs a leader, but what is it that makes the leader a successful health care manager? Management theory recognizes three major approaches to the study of leadership. Each of these approaches takes a slightly different view in an attempt to better understand and predict leadership success. The theories to be studied are the trait, behavioral, and contingency/situational approaches.

The Trait Approach

Common sense tells us that some people may be natural born leaders. Many great leaders such as John Kennedy, Abraham Lincoln, Moses, Mao Tse Tung, and Winston Churchill all seem to have had characteristics or traits that made them somewhat different from everyone else. In some instances, these individuals seemed to have possessed an aura which separated them from their followers. Based on these observations, the first systematic effort by psychologists and other researchers was to identify a set of personal characteristics that separate effective and ineffective leaders. It was believed that once the key traits could be identified (those which all effective leaders possessed), the problem of how to select a leader would be solved. It would simply then be a matter of finding the person with the traits or characteristics and selecting them as the leader.

Although there is considerable support for the idea, researchers have failed to identify leadership traits that can be used consistently for designating individuals as leaders or non-leaders.[8] This is not to imply that individual traits have nothing to do with leadership. Leaders have been found to be somewhat more intelligent, taller, self-confident, and more extroverted than non-leaders. It should be recognized, however, that individual traits must be evaluated in relation to other things. It may be that some leaders become more self-confident once they attain a leadership position. Some traits may be a result, rather than a cause, of an individual's leadership ability.

To discover the research into the trait approach was unable to uncover evidence that clearly distinguishes leaders from non-leaders may be somewhat discouraging. Despite the theory's obvious limitations, it has made significant contributions toward understanding leadership. Many universities, for example, have a department of physical therapy which is run by a physical therapist who has educational experience. Hospitals require physical therapists, nurses and other health care professionals to possess university degrees and be licensed by the state in which they practice. These are considered personal traits or characteristics essential to a profession.

Many managers will argue that individuals who verbalize well, who are slightly more intelligent than their followers, who are socially mature and reasonably self-confident, and are motivated and oriented toward human relations, contain those personal traits which make them more likely to become leaders. Despite the fact that none of these personal traits or characteristics is absolutely necessary to assume a leadership role, they will be of assistance in helping the leader perform effectively.

One trait which is effective in leadership is the motivation to become a leader.[9] The stronger an individual's motivation to become a leader, the more likely the person is to achieve a position of leadership. The effective leader has a high motivational drive and is particularly interested in achieving power and self-actualization over the situations they control.

Behavioral Theory

Once it became apparent that researchers could not isolate a set of personal traits or characteristics of successful leaders, attention shifted to the behavioral leadership theory. The behavioral approach to leadership studies the behavior of leaders by focusing on what leaders do rather than what leaders are.

The initial interest in the behavior of leaders began with research conducted at the University of Michigan and Ohio State University. Researchers conducted a study with small children to determine the effects of autocratic, democratic and laissez-faire leadership on performance.[10]

The autocratic leadership style is evidenced by very tight supervision. This style of leadership is repressive and generally withholds communication from subordinates. The supervisor only communicates when it is necessary for the performance of a job. The members of management make decisions unilaterally without consulting members of the department. Commands are obeyed to avoid being punished.

The democratic leadership style, as used in the study, was a much looser form of supervision. The democratic style permitted the group to discuss relevant matters and make decisions. A democratic style of leadership encourages a free flow of communication among group members. In the research with the children, each child was permitted to work with whomever they chose and received support for their work efforts.

The laissez-faire leader is one who leaves people alone to perform their jobs. There is an absolute minimum of supervision, with the assumption that each person will be self-motivating. The manager does, however, remain available to act as a consultant. The supervisor willingly provides information and guidance but allows the person to arrive at his or her own solution.

The results of the research provided insight as to how each of the three styles affected performance. Those children in the autocratic group produced a greater quantity of work but almost completely stopped working when the leader left the area. Those children supervised by the democratic leader produced a superior quality of work and had only a slight decrease in performance when the leader was absent. The children under the laissez-faire approach did considerably less work, of which was poorer quality than either the democratic or autocratic groups.

As a result of the leadership studies at Ohio State University, the researchers were able to identify three styles of leadership that seem to be of particular importance.[11] The three styles are: supportive, participative, and instrumental leadership. The applications of these are discussed below.

Supportive Leadership

A health care manager who demonstrates a supportive style of leadership shows a high concern for people and a low concern for the task or activity. Supportive leadership considers the needs of subordinates and focuses on warm interpersonal relationships while avoiding conflict and attempting to seek harmony in decision making. A supportive leader assumes an employee desires to do his or her best. As a result of the desire to do their best, the manager will be of assistance in allowing subordinates to achieve their goals. The supportive health care manager will treat subordinates with respect and avoid the use of coercive power. According to the Ohio State researchers, supportive leaders will:

1) Offer to assist subordinates with personal problems.
2) Provide rewards for excellence in performance.
3) Are not overly demanding of employees.
4) Express gratitude and appreciation for a job done well.
5) Try to remain open, friendly, and approachable.

The supportive leader attempts to generate goodwill within the department and organization. Those who adhere to the use of supportive leadership do so because they believe it generates goodwill among employees and leads to higher job satisfaction. Subordinate satisfaction is usually high and turnover low in groups where leaders are rated high in supportiveness.

Participative Leadership

The health care manager who displays participative leadership treats employees as equals and allows them to influence decisions regarding departmental policy and procedure. A participative leader shares information, power, and influence. All subordinates who will be affected by a managerial decision will be given an opportunity to express their opinions and influence the decision. The leader will encourage subordinates to offer suggestions and to be both creative and independent in their own thinking. To accomplish this the manager will:

1) Hold regular staff meetings which provide information of value to subordinates.
2) Actively seek the opinions of subordinates within the department. Physical therapists, assistants, and aides will be encouraged to provide solutions to departmental problems.
3) Avoid the evaluation and final selection of an alternative until the involved parties have had an opportunity to influence the decision.

Participative leadership can be of great assistance to the director of the physical therapy department. Managerial decision making may demonstrate a dramatic improvement because of the added expertise and input of others in the department. Employees who have been provided with an opportunity to influence a managerial decision may begin reporting higher job satisfaction. This is simply because they feel they have more control over the factors which influence their job.

In utilizing the participative style of leadership the health care manager must recognize the importance of two contingency variables. The two variables are the task, or the job the employee is performing, and the characteristics of the individual. When the task is designed so there is little or no opportunity for the employee to become a part of the decision-making process, the participative style is of little value. For example, a physical therapy aide who asks to attend a patient rehabilitation planning session may look upon attendance at the meeting as a waste of time since all decisions will be made by the medical doctors and the physical therapists. On the other hand, an aide who asks to attend a preliminary discussion for developing a design for a new facility may be encouraged if requested to provide input towards designing the department.

The participative leadership style will be most effective when subordinates are predisposed to it and have a high degree of intelligence. The higher the intelligence of the subordinate, the more likely they are to engage in participative decision making. Participative leadership is also conducive to situations where the subordinates have more knowledge about a subject matter than the manager.

Instrumental Leadership

The instrumental style of leadership is characterized by a health care manager who ensures the department reaches its objectives and goals through careful planning, organizing, coordinating, and controlling of subordinate activities. According to the researchers at Ohio State, some of the typical leader behaviors would include:

1) Assignment of specific tasks to employees.
2) Ensuring the worker understands the job.
3) Clearly defined standards of job performance.
4) Work is scheduled for employees.
5) Policies and procedures are followed.

The instrumental style of leadership is often evidenced when there are pressures for output from sources other than the department manager. For example, a hospital administrator may encourage the department director to begin seeing a larger volume of patients. Requests such as these may be for any number of reasons, including such things as a dwindling profit margin. In a situation such as this, the administrator is the outside source who is encouraging greater output.

The instrumental style will be most effective in situations where the personalities of employees are such that they can be told what to do and how to do it. In general, if the employee finds the task or job satisfying they will be more likely to follow established standards of job performance.

The Contingency/Situational Approaches to Leadership

The trait approach to leadership attempted to distinguish leaders from non-leaders by examining the traits or characteristics of successful leaders. The behavioral leadership theory was primarily concerned with what a leader does. The contingency approach to the study of leadership indicates how a manager should behave to lead most effectively. The contingency approach does this by:

1) Identifying factors considered most important under a given set of circumstances.

2) Predicting an appropriate style of leadership that will be most effective when presented with a given set of circumstances.

There are a number of elements in a given situation which will influence the choice of an appropriate leadership style. Some of the factors include time limitations, requisite skill and knowledge, inclinations of the leader and followers, and many other environmental variables. Many of the most recent investigations into the subject of leadership have concluded that no single leadership style is right for every manager. Instead, it is important to recognize the contingency/situational approach. The contingency/situational approach designates the style of leadership to be used when evaluating the situation, the task, the people, the environmental variables, and the individual organization.

The Tannenbaum and Schmidt Model

In 1958, Robert Tannenbaum and Warren Schmidt published an article in an issue of the *Harvard Business Review*. The article was entitled, "How to Choose a Leadership Pattern." This article was so well received by practicing managers and academicians that it was reproduced in 1973 as a "classic."[12] In this article, the authors suggest that managers who are aware of the forces they will face are able to move more rapidly and make the necessary modifications in style to cope with changes in the environment. The three forces which should be considered before choosing a leadership behavior are:

1) Forces in the manager.
2) Forces in the subordinate.
3) Forces in the situation.

The relationship between these forces can be visualized in Figure 4-1. It is important to recognize that the figure does not indicate that either end of the continuum is more effective than the other. The balance between the manager's power and influence in decision making, and that of the subordinates, will be determined by the forces of the manager, the subordinates, and the situation. Each of these will be discussed in the following:

FORCES IN THE MANAGER: The manager's behavior will be influenced by his or her background, knowledge, values and experience.

1) THE VALUE SYSTEM. Does the manager encourage others to participate in decision making? What is the manager's assessment of a fair

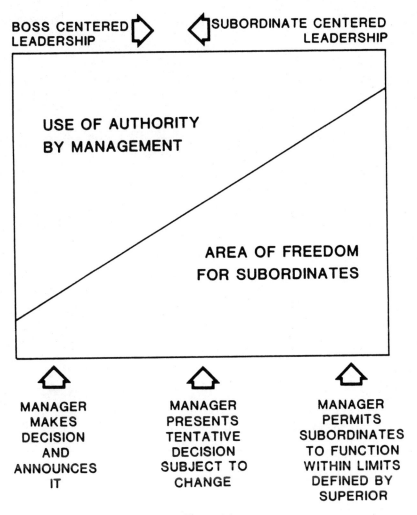

Figure 4-1.

day's work? A health care manager who values individual rights and freedoms often allows greater flexibility in task performance.

2) CONFIDENCE IN EMPLOYEES. Every manager has varying degrees of confidence in an employee's ability to properly perform a job. These attitudes are frequently reflected in the evaluation of the subordinate's performance.

3) TYPE OF LEADERSHIP. There are some managers who are autocratic in their dealings with employees. An autocratic manager is one who wants to direct and control a majority of the actions within

the department. Other managers prefer to allow employees greater freedom and can be classified as more participative in their leadership behavior.

4) SECURITY. Some health care managers have the ability to make a decision and be confident in knowing the possible ramifications that may result from the decision. Other managers feel as though much is to be gained from keeping everyone informed. Security is the confidence the individual has in his or her decision-making ability and the tolerance for unpredictable behaviors of participating subordinates.

FORCES IN THE SUBORDINATES: Managers must also consider forces in the subordinates before selecting an appropriate leadership style. There are a large number of forces which can potentially influence a subordinate's personality. Each subordinate has a unique set of expectations concerning the level of decision making they like, responsibility desired, and what they expect from management. Subordinates will also differ in the degree to which they identify with the organization's objectives and goals. It is the manager's responsibility to understand the particular needs, desires, and career objectives of their employees.

FORCES IN THE SITUATION: Within the organization there are a number of situational forces which will determine a manager's leadership effectiveness. Some of the forces to be considered are the organization, the effectiveness of the group, the tasks to be performed, the influence of time, and relevant environmental forces affecting the organization.

1) THE ORGANIZATION. All health care organizations have values which are demonstrated by action and communicated by policy. The values important to the organization will influence the style of leadership adopted. The values adopted by top management are also likely to be seen in lower levels of management.

2) THE EFFECTIVENESS OF THE GROUP. In most hospital settings groups are divided by function. The physical therapy department is an example of a group established by function for the purpose of providing rehabilitative services. Groups which work well together, and accomplish goals, will be given more autonomy to perform than those which are recognized as being ineffective.

3) TASKS PERFORMED. The assigned task has a great deal to do with an employee's job satisfaction. If the group finds the task rewarding, they will be more likely to be satisfied with their jobs than a group

who has been delegated a task which cannot be successfully accomplished. Assigning tasks which cannot be successfully completed leads to eventual frustration, poor attitudes, and perhaps turnover or absenteeism.

4) TIME. Increasingly, time is of the essence. When the health care manager has only a few moments to make a decision, it is not always possible to involve others in the decision-making process. When time is not a factor, the manager may discover that the participative style of leadership is appropriate.

5) ENVIRONMENTAL VARIABLES. The health care manager cannot make decisions based solely upon the internal environment of the organization. The external environment of the organization consists of a number of factors, including the political climate of a community, suppliers, the federal government, and how consumers feel about the health care services offered by the organization.

Interestingly enough, many health care managers adopt a style of leadership that closely parallels that of their own superior. If the superior reflects an open style of management and encourages the use of human relations, the subordinate manager may perform likewise. If the superior is decisive, the subordinate manager may follow the same leadership style and become more task oriented.

The most important aspect of selecting a leadership style is for the manager to choose one which is comfortable for them and appropriate for the subordinates and the work situation. The best leaders are flexible. They continually evaluate their own position, the changes occurring within the subordinates, the situation, and then make informed decisions. Those health care managers who achieve the best results recognize that the chances of meeting desired levels of performance are improved if their leadership style reflects an optimal balance of the forces of the manager, the subordinate and the situation.

Fiedler's Contingency Theory

The contingency model of leadership, developed by Fred Fiedler, emphasizes the importance of the situation in leadership effectiveness.[13] The model postulates that performance of a group depends upon the leader's style and the relative favorableness of the situation for the leader. A leader may select a style that can range from highly task oriented to highly relationship oriented. The favorableness in a situation is determined by three major dimensions. They are:

- Leader/member relations
- Leader position power
- Task structure

Leader/member relations refers to the leader's evaluation of being accepted by the group. If the leader feels as though he or she gets along well with the group and the group respects the leader, then the leader is less likely to rely on formal authority to get the job done. If the manager is disliked, he or she may have to rely on orders to get subordinates to accomplish their assigned tasks.

Leader position power is the scope of the leader's power base. As presented earlier, power is an interesting form of influence which can be exercised in many ways. Here, power is referred to as the degree to which the leader possesses legitimate reward and coercive power to influence the behavior of subordinates.

Task structure is the extent to which a task is routine (structured) or complex (unstructured). A task which is routine will have clearly defined instructions on how it should be performed and what goals are to be achieved. For example, a department supervisor may have clearly established policies and procedures for the scheduling of a new patient. In a situation such as this, the manager will possess a great deal of authority since there are clear guidelines by which to measure performance. If, however, the task is complex and non-routine, the leader may have little or no more knowledge than the subordinate about the situation. When there are no clear guidelines on how to proceed, group members can more easily question or disagree with the leader's instructions.

There are several important implications which can be derived from the Fiedler model. First, when the situation is either highly favorable or highly unfavorable for the leader the most effective style of leadership will be task oriented. When there is a good group atmosphere, the leader's position power is high and the task is structured, the situation is highly favorable. If, however, the task is unstructured, the leader lacks group support and has little position power, a task-motivated leadership is the only hope for achieving the primary goal of the group. A classification of situational favorableness is provided in Figure 4-2.

The relationship-motivated leadership style is recommended when the situation tends to be neither favorable or unfavorable. Referring

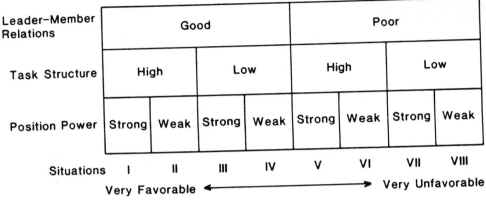

Figure 4-2.

again to Figure 4-2, the leader obtains the best group efficiency in situations in which the task is structured but the leader is disliked and must evidence concern for subordinates. The leader also obtains the best group efficiency when the leader is liked but the group has an unstructured task and the leader must depend on the willingness and creativity of the group to accomplish goals.

The Fiedler model of leadership has been the subject of a growing body of research which has failed to neither verify or refute the Fiedler model.[14] It has, however, proven to be a significant addition to the study of leadership. The Fiedler model has drawn attention to the importance of considering other factors that can affect the leader's attempt to influence the behavior of subordinates. As such, the model serves to illustrate how a manager's leadership style can be effective in one situation and not effective in others.

Situational Leadership and the Life Cycle Theory

The situational leadership theory developed by Paul Hersey and Kenneth H. Blanchard has also been referred to as the life cycle theory of leadership.[15] The theory is situational, as is Fiedler's, except for one major difference. The theory emphasizes that the leader must use an adaptive style of leadership based on a diagnosis of the situation. Accordingly, a leader's strategy and behavior should be situational based primarily on the maturity or immaturity of the followers. The theory is illustrated in Figure 4-3.

The maturity continuum for subordinates is divided into three stages. These are indicated in Figure 4-3 as low, average, and high maturity.

The Life Cycle Theory

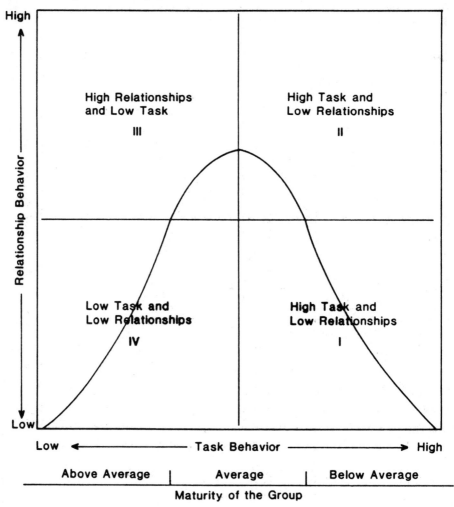

Figure 4-3.

The theory proposes that the leader, to be effective, must change leadership styles as the subordinates gain additional maturity. If the leader has followers who are low in maturity, the leader should adopt a style of behavior as is indicated in quadrant one. As the followers increase in maturity, the sequence of leader behavior should change accordingly. The changes the leader would be required to follow are indicated in quadrants two, three, and four of Figure 4-3.

The authors define maturity not as a function of age or emotional stability but as a willingness to accept responsibility and the desire for achievement. The authors also believe the leader must consider the individual's educational background, experience, and task-related ability. The maturity variables should be considered only in relation to the specific task which is to be performed, not to the individual as a whole.

Task behavior is the extent to which the leader must organize and explain the activities necessary for subordinates to accomplish. This includes explaining what each is to do in order to complete an entire job. To do this requires the manager establish well-defined channels of communication and organization.

The relationship between the manager and the subordinate moves through four phases or quadrants. These four phases take on the appearance of a normal life cycle as would be seen in the field of marketing. As subordinates change in levels of maturity, the manager will also need to change in order to be effective. To use the chart, the manager must first determine the maturity level of the group and then trace a line upward until it intercepts the curved line in one of the four quadrants. That intersection and the number in the quadrant will represent the most effective leadership style.

In the initial phase (high task and low relationship) the manager will emphasize performing the job-related activity. A group of new employees in a physical therapy department will initially be introduced to a job through formal policies, procedures, and methods of patient care. The manager will, of course, be friendly but tend to emphasize acquainting the employees to the organization and to the tasks to be performed.

Once the new employees become acquainted with the organization and their tasks, the health care manager may begin to implement the more relationship-motivated behavior as seen in quadrant two. It remains essential, however, to continue to emphasize high task behavior, since the employee remains unwilling or unable to accept full responsibility for the task. In the process of initiating relationship behavior, the manager may begin to express increasing trust and confidence in the work the employees are performing.

In the third phase it will be inappropriate for the health care manager to be directive. Employee maturity, ability and achievement motivation have increased. At this point the employee knows the patient treatment tasks which are to be performed and will resent a high task oriented leadership style. Throughout this period the manager should continue to maintain a high relationship with subordinates by being considerate and supportive.

The fourth phase is characterized by employees who are confident and experienced. They are, for the most part, self-directed. Upon reaching this stage, subordinates are considered mature and no longer need or desire a directive style of leadership from the manager. Subordinates know their tasks and perform them without managerial encouragement.

The theory as presented by Hersey and Blanchard is quite promising. It assumes that today's employees are more educated, technically competent, and more highly motivated than ever before. For the health care manager, the theory does indeed have application. If, for example, the director of physical therapy desires to add a cardiac rehabilitation unit to the present facility it will require careful planning and direction in order to be successful. In the initial stages of implementation, the manager may have to guide subordinates by presenting a high task, low relationship leadership style until they become familiar with the cardiac rehabilitation policies, procedures and methods of organization. As the unit becomes more established and the subordinates become more mature, the leadership style should change and become less directive and more relationship oriented. The key to managerial success with this leadership theory is that subordinates must continually be assessed to determine which style of leader behavior will be the most appropriate.

HEALTH CARE LEADERSHIP:
SOME THOUGHTS ON MANAGERIAL ACTION

As a result of reading this chapter it has probably become readily apparent that there are a number of conflicting theories regarding how to become a successful leader. Is there any one style that is best? The answer is probably not. There are a number of situational, personal and group variables that influence leadership effectiveness and, as such, make it almost impossible for the leader to be totally autocratic, democratic, participative, or considerate. There are, however, some guidelines which can be followed to increase the chances for success in health care management.

In order to be successful in a management position requiring leadership, the individual must have a good self-awareness. The leader must be able to diagnose his or her style of leadership, listing the positive and negative traits and characteristics possessed. What style of leadership do you project? Do your subordinates view the same style of leadership or do they view you as possibly manipulative? A self-analysis of one's psychological, sociological, and physiological makeup will be essential for the physical therapist who desires to demonstrate leadership effectiveness.

The health care manager must also depend heavily on developing diagnostic skills to assess the maturity, expectations, skills, and cohesiveness of the work group. The job of the leader is to diagnose potential group problems, propose solutions, and remove obstacles to the attainment of individual and group goals. Only by understanding what motivates the group can the leader develop plans to reward group members and guide future performance.

Is the image of the strong, silent type who speaks few words but leaves no doubt who is in charge an accurate portrayal of a leader? Research into that theory fails to confirm the view. In many cases, research has indicated the opposite situation exists; namely, the higher the individual's verbal output, the more likely they are to be viewed as a leader.[16] For the health care manager, these findings indicate that the leader must be willing to lead discussions, encourage involvement and contribute ideas to be more recognized as a group leader. In health care, as well as in the world of business, silence does not cultivate the image of a leader.

Finally, it is important for the leader to remain as consistent as possible in order to be perceived as being effective. Former President Jimmy Carter was only the third president in ninety-six years to be turned away from office by the American public when he was defeated for re-election in 1980. Although a great number of factors contributed to his political defeat, lack of consistency was named as a significant factor. Author E.J. Hughes stated: "The American people find it easy to forgive a leader's great mistakes, but not long meanderings."[17] To be an effective leader, the physical therapist must consider all options which are available, choose a course of action, and stick with the selection. For many health care professionals, consistency represents stability and is, therefore, important to being viewed as a leader.

REFERENCES

1. Robert B. Cattell, "New Concepts for Measuring Leadership in Terms of Group Syntality," Human Relations (1951), pp. 161–184.
2. Chris Argyris, "Leadership, Learning, and Changing the Status Quo," Organizational Dynamics (Winter 1976).

3. Robert Dubin, Human Relations in Administration (Englewood Cliffs, NJ: Prentice-Hall, 1951).

4. Ralph M. Stogdill, Handbook of Leadership (New York: Free Press, 1974).

5. David C. McClelland and David H. Burnham, "Power is the Great Motivator," Harvard Business Review, Vol. 54 (March–April 1976), pp. 100–110.

6. John R. P. French and Bertram Raven, "The Bases of Social Power," in Dorwin Cartwright and A. F. Zander, eds., Group Dynamics, 2nd ed. (Evanston, IL: Row, Peterson, 1960), pp. 607–623.

7. Douglas McGregor, The Human Side of Enterprises (New York: McGraw-Hill, 1960). pp. 33–48.

8. R. Stogdill, op., cit., p. 9.

9. E. Ghiselli, Explorations in Managerial Talent (Pacific Palisades, CA: Wordsworth Publishing Company, 1971).

10. R. White and R. Lippet, "Leader Behavior and Member Reaction in Three Social Climates," In Group Dynamics: Research and Theory, 3rd ed. D. Cartwright and A. Zander, (eds.) Harper & Row, 1967, pp. 318–336.

11. C. Schriesheim and S. Kerr, "Theories and Measures of Leadership: A Critical Appraisal of Current and Future Directions," In Leadership: The Cutting Edge. J. Hunt and L. Larson, (eds.) Carbondale IL: Southern Illinois University Press, 1977, pp. 9–45, 51–56.

12. Robert Tannenbaum and Warren H. Schmidt, "How to Choose a Leadership Pattern," Harvard Business Review, May–June 1973, pp. 162–180.

13. Fred F. Fiedler, A Theory of Leadership Effectiveness (New York: McGraw-Hill, 1967).

14. D. Hosking and C. Schrieheim, "Review Essay," Administrative Science Quarterly, 23, 1978, 496–505; and C. Schrieheim and S. Kerr, "Theories and Measures of Leadership: A Critical Appraisal of Current and Future Directions," In Leadership: The Cutting Edge, J. Hunt and L. Larson (eds.) Carbondale, IL: Southern Illinois University Press, 1977, pp. 9–45, 51–56. See also R. Rice, "Leader LPC and Follower Satisfaction: A Review," Organizational Behavior and Human Performance, 28, 1981, 1–25.

15. Paul Hersey and Kenneth H. Blanchard, Management of Organizational Behavior, 3d ed. (Englewood Cliffs, NJ: Prentice-Hall, 1977), p. 161.

16. E. I. Hollander & J. W. Julian, "A Further Look at Leader Legitimacy, Influence, and Innovation," in L. Berkowitz (ed.), Group Processes, (New York: Academic Press, 1978), and R. M. Sorrentino & R. G. Boutillier, "The Effect of Quantity and Quality of Verbal Interaction on Ratings of Leadership Ability," Journal of Experimental Social Psychology, 1975, 11, pp. 403–411.

17. E. J. Hughes, "The Presidency Versus Jimmy Carter," Fortune, December 4, 1978, p. 58.

Chapter Five

MANAGERIAL COMMUNICATION

One important ingredient of effective health care management is the ability to communicate with others. As a health care supervisor you will soon discover that your ability to communicate will determine your overall success as a department manager. Communication is fundamental to the managerial activities of organizing, decision making, motivation, leadership, and to achieving a coordination of services. A health care manager is required to gather information from others, issue appropriate directives, and ensure everyone has a thorough understanding of what is to be accomplished. The most effective health care managers are those who have mastered the ability to communicate.

Consider your present position as a health care supervisor. Is there any one area of departmental operation or patient treatment that could be performed without some form of communication? The answer to this question is obviously not. As a supervisor it is very likely you will spend as much as 80 percent of your day either receiving or sending valuable information to supervisors, subordinates, patients, or physicians. Communication is regarded as so important that the readers of the *Harvard Business Review* chose "the ability to communicate" as an executive's most essential qualification for promotion to higher levels.[1]

In your career as a health care professional, you have undoubtedly worked with a supervisor who demonstrated excellent clinical skills, was knowledgeable and easy to work with but for some reason never seemed to get anything accomplished. Quite often the supervisor had well-developed plans but for some reason they were never communicated to the members of the department. The reason they were never communicated was because the supervisor lacked the necessary skills to ensure all members had a thorough understanding of what was to be accomplished. Communication makes it possible for others to understand the manager's desires and intentions. The ability to communicate is a skill. Exercising the managerial responsibility of leadership is impossible without communication. To be an effective health care manager the skill must continually be practiced. Only through practice can the physical therapist learn to motivate, lead, and coordinate the activities of the department toward desired objectives and goals.

COMMUNICATION IN THE HEALTH CARE ENVIRONMENT

Communication in health care is the process by which information and understanding is passed from one individual to another. To communicate simply means to make oneself clearly understood by others. If the message is not clear or not fully understood, communication has not taken place. Where communication is incomplete the result will be errors and confusion. When the communication process breaks down or is incomplete, the risks to the patient can increase dramatically.

The most important concept to be understood in the definition of communication is that the process involves two or more people. One person is the sender of the message and the other is the receiver. A message cannot be communicated unless there is an individual to receive it. For example, a letter which has been typed and mailed has not been communicated until it is read and understood by the receiver. A supervisor who is unhappy with a subordinate's performance cannot expect a change in behavior until the dissatisfaction is communicated directly to the subordinate.

Another important aspect of the definition of communication is that of understanding. Each person is endowed with certain capacities for understanding. For communication to be effective there must be an understanding between the two individuals involved. If the message received by the individual is the same as the one which was intended, then it can be said that a communication has taken place. If there is a lack of understanding on the part of the receiver, then only written or spoken information has been relayed.

An effective communications network is needed between the administration and subordinates of an organization. Effective communication allows the development and administration of policies and procedures. When misunderstandings arise concerning the exact meaning of a policy or procedure, the manager must clarify the area of concern. The ultimate success of the health care manager is based upon the ability to communicate with subordinates. Just as a physical therapist must learn to skillfully communicate with patients, so must the health care manager communicate with department members.

THE CHANNELS OF COMMUNICATION IN HEALTH CARE ORGANIZATIONS

Within every health care organization there are two recognized channels of communication. The first channel is based on the structure of the organization and is called the formal channel. The second channel of communication is known as the informal channel. Each channel will carry vital, and sometimes not so vital, messages in either upward, downward, lateral, or diagonal directions.

The Formal Channel of Communication

The structure of the health care organization will ultimately determine the formal channel of communication. When the structure of the organization is initially established a network of authority relationships is also determined. As such, the formal channel of communication extends from the chief administrator of the organization down to the lowest level. Information will flow upward, downward, laterally, or diagonally within the formal channels of communication. At each level, administrative and non-administrative personnel will be called to act upon the information which has been provided. The formal channel will follow the hierarchial structure of the health care organization (Figure 5-1).

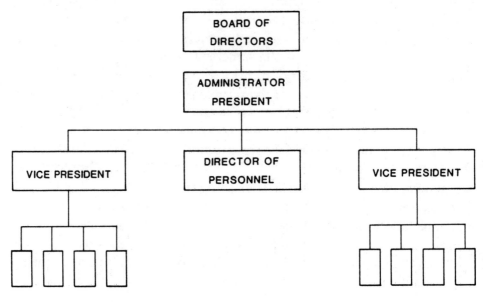

Figure 5-1.

Downward Communication

In the hospital setting the downward channel of communication is used specifically by members of management for sending information to employees at lower levels in the health care organization. Information included in the downward channel will involve the issuance of directives, goals, policies and memorandums. There are primarily five reasons why managers use the downward form of communication.[2]

1) TO ISSUE JOB INSTRUCTIONS. Management often desires to provide information concerning how a job should be performed as well as what results are expected.

2) JOB RATIONALE. Whenever a new position or service is created in an organization the manager may find it necessary to explain the job and its purpose to others.

3) FOR DESCRIPTIVE PURPOSES. The manager may use downward communication for describing policies, rules, regulations, and the benefits provided by the organization.
4) TO PROVIDE FEEDBACK. A manager will frequently use downward communication to provide feedback concerning individual job performance.
5) FOR INDOCTRINATION PURPOSES. Top management may stress the importance of employee involvement in certain events favorable to the organization. Employees may, for example, be encouraged to devote time or contribute monies to certain charitable community organizations.

Downward communication is probably one of the most frequently used methods of managerial communication in the health care organization. Downward communication serves to link each level of the organization's hierarchy in a coordinated fashion. Upon receiving downward communication, the manager assumes the responsibility for seeing that the information reaches its final destination (Figure 5-2).

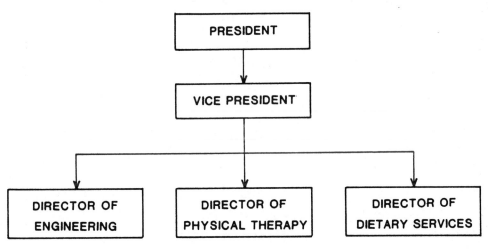

Figure 5-2.

Upward Communication

In most health care organizations downward communication is recognized as being directive, whereas upward communication is considered informative. The director of physical therapy has the responsibility of keeping his or her immediate supervisor informed of the activities occurring within the department. This includes informing the immediate supervisor of changing personnel requirements, problems with department operation, or providing suggestions on how to alter or improve the quality of health care provided by the organization.

In all health care organizations top, middle, and lower level management must openly encourage upward communication. Subordinates must be made to feel as though they can express their ideas and opinions on all work-related matters. To encourage upward communication management should express interest in obtaining all facts relevant to the operation of the organization. By expressing interest in obtaining vital information the manager is attempting to avoid a situation whereby a subordinate builds up frustration or hostility over a matter which easily could have been prevented. When employees feel their messages are not valued by the members of management they may seek other outlets by which to vent their anger or frustration (Figure 5-3).

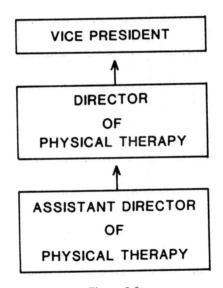

Figure 5-3.

When the health care manager receives vital information from subordinates he or she must respond in an appropriate fashion. Significant findings should be reported to the next level of management as soon as they become known. Department directors can suffer a personal loss of credibility if top management discovers important information through another channel. In some situations your supervisor may have to react quickly to the information provided. It is, therefore, essential to gather all the facts, ascertain their immediate relevancy, and pass them on to your supervisor.

When presenting information to your supervisor always try to be objective and straightforward. This may be partially difficult in negative situations, since no one wants to tarnish their image in front of management. In some situations it may appear advantageous to "soften" unpleasant information so as to lessen the blow. Eventually, once the next level of management has a chance to investigate, the full extent of the problem will become known. Therefore, always try to remain objective and present the facts as they are known, even if it means taking personal responsibility for a mistake that has been made.

Lateral Communication

Lateral communication is used extensively in the health care setting as well as in business and industry. This form of communication occurs most often between people and departments who are on the same organizational level but who perform different functions. The director of physical therapy may, for example, communicate with the director of occupational therapy concerning a patient or an organizational problem.

Lateral communication is especially important in health care, since it helps to ensure the members of the organization work together towards accomplishing objectives and goals. When two departments fail to communicate, it is the patient who has the most to lose. One of the primary functions of a health care manager is to ensure communication between departments does not break down. Lateral communication is graphically portrayed in Figure 5-4.

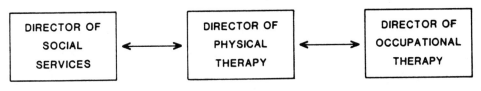

Figure 5-4.

Diagonal Communication

The diagonal direction of communication involves the flow of messages from one individual or group to another individual or group not on the same lateral plane within the health care organization. The director of nursing may, for example, speak with one of the staff physical therapists concerning the level of care a patient is receiving or some of the services offered by the department. Here, the intent may not be to bypass the director of physical therapy but instead to perform a more direct communication link.

Diagonal communication of this type serves to integrate the various allied health care services. One way for the director of physical therapy to promote the department and the profession is to actively engage in diagonal communications with all personnel in the hospital setting. This can be accomplished by providing presentations to each department and addressing the goals of rehabilitative services (Figure 5-5).

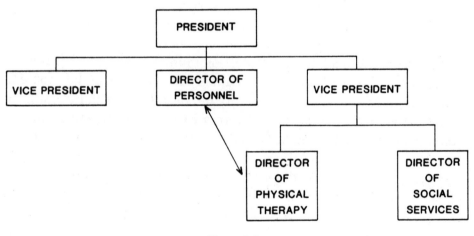

Figure 5-5.

Informal Communication Channels:
The Workings Of The Grapevine

The most commonly recognized system of communication within a health care organization is that of the formal channel of communication. As previously noted, the formal channel develops directly from the design of the organization and follows the established hierarchial pattern.

The informal channel, commonly referred to as the grapevine because of its haphazard and irregular pattern of movement, develops in all organizations as an outgrowth of the desire for people to interact socially and communicate with one another.

Although organizations strive to develop sound formal channels of communication, it should be understood that the grapevine will evolve as a purely natural activity. The contacts which occur between employees at all levels within the organization encourage the development of spontaneous channels of communication. Through these channels information will be passed up, down, laterally, and diagonally. The information passed will consist of both rumor and fact.

The grapevine provides important functions within the health care organization. First, it serves to fulfill the individual's desire to be kept "in the know" about fellow health care professionals, patients, nurses, doctors, and many others. Second, the grapevine provides members of the organization with an opportunity to speculate on possible activities or events to occur in the future. The informal channel can be of assistance in relieving apprehensions about potential changes in a department or organization as well as providing individuals with an outlet for their imagination.

As health care professionals, all of us have been part of the grapevine at one time or another. The amount of involvement a health care member will have in the grapevine will vary, although some people are more active participants than others. The grapevine holds no stable membership, nor does it follow a definitive pattern. An individual may be active in the grapevine on one occasion and be absent in another. As supervisors, it is important to recognize the type and content of the information transmitted through the grapevine. Valuable insights can be obtained concerning subordinate attitudes, feelings, and concerns.

Managerial Uses for the Grapevine

The information which passes through the grapevine is rarely 100 percent accurate. Much of the information is distorted, half correct, or based solely on the private interpretations, conjecture and suspicions of a few individuals. A majority of the organization's employees will listen to at least some of the information carried in the grapevine, but few will pass it along. As a manager who is observing the workings of the grapevine it will soon become apparent that some members are more active participants than others. Many of the most active participants engage in the grapevine because they feel their prestige is somehow enhanced by knowing and disseminating the latest information. These same individuals may willingly alter some of the information, since they know they cannot be held accountable for the information and origins of the rumor. As such, many employees feel surprisingly comfortable as active participants in the workings of the grapevine.

Although the grapevine does carry a considerable amount of inaccurate information, it can still be beneficial to the health care organization and its managers. The director of physical therapy is often tempted to eliminate the grapevine, since it carries so much misinformation. Eliminating the grapevine is next to impossible. The fact is, the supervisor could no more eliminate the grapevine than he or she could eliminate the formal organization. The supervisor of physical therapy must accept the informal channel of communication and look for ways it can be used for managerial advantage. Utilizing the grapevine for managerial advantage requires the supervisor to first determine who is spreading most of the information. Only when the manager knows the origins of a message can the grapevine be used for managerial advantage.

The rumors and misinformation which circulate throughout the organization may be as a result of a number of underlying factors. Employees will often engage in the rumor-spreading process as a result of wishful thinking, fear, or in an effort to disrupt the organization or one of its members. An employee may, for example, desperately desire a raise and begin spreading rumors which indicate management is in the process of preparing to increase everyone's salary by 7 percent. As supervisor, it is important to recognize that rumors such as these can have a devastating effect on department morale if it turns out to be false. When presented with a situation such as this, management must move quickly to set the record straight. If top management has no plans to offer a raise, the supervisor should conduct a meeting which tactfully denies the possibility. Moving rapidly to dispel a rumor will be less traumatic to department morale than allowing employees to discover the truth after a long waiting period resulting from managerial inaction.

When a rumor is circulated based on fear, the manager must, once again, move quickly to correct the misinformation. If, for example, the hospital has had a prolonged period of declining utilization, budgetary requirements may call for a reduction in the size of the hospital's staff. Once the members of top management announce a reduction in staff, the grapevine will immediately circulate rumors and misinformation as to who will be released from employment. If the director of physical therapy has been advised as to how the cutbacks will affect the department, all employees should immediately be notified. If cutbacks are projected, advise those individuals most likely to be terminated so they can make plans for future employment.

There may be situations where a rumor is circulating which the supervisor can neither confirm nor deny simply because of a lack of information or knowledge concerning the subject matter. When confronted with this problem, the supervisor should contact the next level of management and discuss the issue that is of concern to employees. If the next level of management indicates the rumor is true, the department manager must inquire as to how much information may be disseminated to employees and when it should be done. In departments which have an assistant director of physical therapy, always meet first with that individual before conducting a meeting with subordinates.

Rumors may also arise as a result of a personal dislike for the director of physical therapy or for the organization. When events such as this occur, the supervisor should attempt to locate the source of the dissatisfaction and meet with the individuals directly involved. All meetings should be held in the privacy of the supervisor's office. Your effectiveness as supervisor will be based upon the respect subordinates have for you as a person. Employees must recognize your sincerity in trying to make the department a good place to work. The more employees believe in you as a leader, the less likely they are to believe a malicious rumor about you or the organization.

METHODS OF COMMUNICATION

There are a number of methods a supervisor may utilize to communicate within the health care organization. Proper use of all methods of communication is the most effective tool the manager has for building and maintaining a well-functioning team of health care professionals. The fact that a supervisor is continually engaged in communication with subordinates does not guarantee that messages are being sent and received properly. Undoubtedly, the spoken word is one of the most important means a supervisor utilizes to communicate. Words, however, are not the only media by which supervisors, physicians, employees, and patients communicate. The modern health care supervisor may also use pictures or actions to further demonstrate the meaning of what is communicated.

Pictures

Every physical therapy department is equipped with pamphlets, pictures, anatomical drawings and models which may be used to explain a diagnosis or treatment method to a patient. For subordinates, pictures or drawings can be used to further increase understanding concerning the proper methods of transferring a patient, body mechanics, or general departmental safety procedures. When subordinates lack a clear understanding of what is being communicated, the use of pictures or drawings will be quite effective in the clarification process.

Actions

As supervisor, many of your actions will be carefully scrutinized by those within and outside of the department. The messages communicated non-verbally will often speak much louder than words. Certain gestures, body movements, a partial smile or frown all communicate meanings to those who work closely with you. In patient care, as well as in health care management, the supervisor must always be aware of facial expressions or actions that imply unintended meanings which result in unintended consequences.

Lack of managerial action or inaction is also a form of communication. The physical therapist who repeatedly takes no action on matters considered important to subordinates communicates a non-verbal message that he or she is indecisive or uncaring. In most instances it is better to take some form of action rather than taking no action at all. Employees are likely to forgive an error in managerial judgment much sooner than they will forget an important decision that a manager did not take the time to make.

It is also important for the manager to avoid displaying reckless behavior or unexplained actions. Emotional outbursts of temper should be avoided. Employees expect a stable departmental environment and desire consistency and fairness in supervision. The manager should not, for example, remove a piece of rehabilitative equipment from the department without first announcing why the equipment is no longer to be used. Unexplained actions and haphazard managerial behavior often communicates feelings of insecurity to employees. This is not to say you must always consult your employees prior to making a decision. It is simply a matter of providing an environment that is consistent and allows employees to know where they stand and what can be expected in the future.

Written and Oral Communication

The importance of using proper written and oral communication in the health care environment is easily understood. Instructions to employees must be clear and specific if the department and the health care organization are to reach designated objectives and goals. You may be familiar with the story in which the supervisor asked the new employee to thoroughly clean and disinfect the whirlpool. Upon return, the supervisor discovered the employee had cleaned the outside of the whirlpool but left the water remaining from the last patient treatment. When questioned as to why the inside of the tub was not cleaned, the employee responded, "I didn't think we should throw out all that perfectly good water."

Words, both written and spoken, represent different meanings to each of us. Many factors influence how an individual interprets a message including such things as training and experience. In any communication process the supervisor must consider the background of the individual to whom the message is intended. Communicating with a new employee is often more time consuming than communicating with an established professional. All forms of communication must carefully consider the particular makeup of the prospective audience.

Health care supervisors often rely extensively on the use of oral communication. It is, of course, much easier to use and more rapid than delivering a handwritten or typed message. Oral communication will allow the physical therapist to discuss a wider variety of topics than would be possible when using the written form of communication. In contrast to the written form of communication, oral messages last only for a moment and can frequently be misunderstood by the receiver. Therefore, when it is considered important to make a permanent record of the communication, the written form should be utilized.

Physical therapy departments often use the written form of communication when the subject matter must be repeatedly reviewed or studied for long periods of time. Policies, procedures, and other methods of department organization are frequently recorded in writing. Patients also receive printed material containing lists of exercises or precautions to take to protect a surgical fixation. Whenever an audience must have specific instruction, written communication helps to ensure better understanding and compliance.

Oral communication is the most extensively relied upon form of communication in the health care environment. Physicians rely on oral communication to transmit treatment orders to both allied personnel and patients. The physical therapist also extensively utilizes oral communication to communicate with patients, physicians, fellow professionals, and supportive personnel. The physical therapist in private practice utilizes oral communication during speaking engagements to promote the services offered by the practice.

Due to the widespread dependence on oral communication, the supervisor should recognize the four advantages derived from becoming skilled in the ability to communicate. First, if done properly, no form of written communication can surpass the use of oral communication. Especially when utilizing face-to-face communication, the skilled supervisor can exchange information, express opinions, or provide motivational stimuli to enhance employee performance.

Second, the oral form of communication provides the opportunity for the therapist to be seen and heard. Written communication can provide detailed information, but patients and fellow health care professionals like to be in an atmosphere which provides visual stimuli. Oral communication provides an opportunity to ask for additional explanations through the open exchange of opinions and ideas.

Third, oral communication allows the supervisor to obtain feedback. When messages are communicated to employees in writing, the supervisor has little or no opportunity to obtain feedback concerning the impact the subject matter had on employee motivation and morale. The use of oral communication also allows the examination of the receiver's facial expressions. A subordinate's response to a supervisory message, both verbal and non-verbal, will indicate whether the intended message was received and understood.

Finally, the supervisor must recognize the importance of communicating in the proper atmosphere. Outside interference can hinder the communication process. The supervisor should select an appropriate time and place in which to communicate with subordinates. A controversial subject should not be discussed at the end of the day or on a Friday. Supervisors must set aside enough time to discuss a subject so employees will not feel hurried or be anxious to leave.

BREAKDOWNS IN THE COMMUNICATION PROCESS

Every health care professional has, at one time or another, witnessed a breakdown in communication. In most situations the breakdown in communication creates nothing more than a minor inconvenience which has no long-lasting side effects. In more extreme cases, breakdowns in communication can be costly to patients or to the organization and its workers.

One of the functions the supervisor of physical therapy must perform is to ensure there is a complete and effective channel of communication established within and outside of the organization. Establishing a communication network requires the manager remain aware of how problems can develop and how they can be prevented. In the health care environment breakdowns in communication can be grouped into three broad categories. The breakdowns may be due to: language, status or position, and the resistance to change.

Breakdowns in Communication Due to Language

You may have heard the phrase "what we have is a failure to communicate." This phrase is often very appropriate in the health care environment where professionals and patients come from diverse backgrounds of training, experience, and knowledge of the medical profession. Physicians are often accused of speaking a language which is totally "alien" to patients. As a result, the physical therapist is frequently left "holding the bag" when it comes to explaining the ramifications of a diagnosis, treatment, or prospective rehabilitative result.

The physical therapist who embarks into health care management soon discovers the position requires use of the language of the profession, the administrator, and the lay person. For example, when the hospital administration speaks of "profits" they are referring to an essential ingredient for ensuring the continued survival of the organization. On the other hand, an employee may regard a "profit" as an excess sum of money that should be returned to the worker in the form of higher wages or benefits. Once in a management position, the language of the therapist is likely to change and begin reflecting the added responsibilities of the assignment.

In order to prevent breakdowns in communication due to language, the supervisor must speak in a manner the receiver understands and can identify with. To accomplish this frequently requires the manager to consider the audience and use the language which is direct and uncomplicated. Remember, the receiver will interpret the language you use based on their own knowledge and frame of reference. Do not automatically assume the individual will interpret the message as you originally intended. If the person has to struggle to interpret what is communicated, they will either become frustrated or disinterested. In either case they will be unlikely to ask questions but rather to fill in the blanks based on their own understanding.

Breakdowns in Communication Due to Status or Position

The modern health care organization contains a number of hierarchial positions occupied by individuals who have varying degrees of responsibility and status. The responsibilities and level of status each person possesses has been conferred by the organization and its management. There is, for example, a profound difference in decision-making authority and responsibility between the chief executive officer and a vice-president. Between hierarchial levels, the type and form of communication will change along with member social interaction. Whenever there is hierarchial distance established between levels of management or between workers, the opportunity exists for communication problems to develop.

The physical therapist striving to become an effective communicator will soon realize that breakdowns in communication due to status or position are the results of individual differences in opinion, negative feelings, or a general lack of interest. Each message delivered by a member of management will be evaluated by the subordinate based on the individual's socioeconomic background and experience. To become an effective communicator, the supervisor must endeavor to visualize how a message will be interpreted from the subordinate's point of view. By doing so, the supervisor can carefully analyze and anticipate the subordinate's response before the message is delivered.

When presenting any message, the supervisor must give careful attention to gestures, smiles, or other facial expressions. Subordinates quickly learn to recognize the underlying meaning of what is being said by carefully examining the supervisor's facial expressions. It is difficult for subordinates to separate what has been said from the manner in which the message was delivered. It is, therefore, essential to communicate in a manner that utilizes the proper mix of gestures to coincide with the intended message.

Resistance to Change

For many, thoughts of change, especially in the work environment, are not welcome intellectual endeavors. In most instances we resist change simply because we are creatures of habit who, if given the opportunity, would like to maintain the status quo. The process of change may be uncomfortable, requiring the learning of new ideas and approaches to patient care. As a result, any message which imparts change for the subordinate may be met with apprehension or suspicion. This is especially true if the message is in conflict with the individual's values or beliefs.

How can a supervisor handle the concerns a subordinate has about change and still encourage the implementation of new ideas and processes? The following provides some managerial recommendations:

1) DEVELOP THE IDEA THAT CHANGE IS GOOD AND PART OF THE PROCESS OF INDIVIDUAL AND ORGANIZATIONAL GROWTH. Communicate to employees that the health care environment is a dynamic and rapidly changing part of the American society. The changes which are occurring require each member to adopt new ideas, methods, and procedures for doing their job. Encourage the belief that change is good and is expected by the health care organization.

2) PROVIDE OPPORTUNITIES FOR SUBORDINATE INTERACTION. Some of the best ways to introduce change is to allow it to develop as an outflow of subordinate interaction. Encourage members to participate in staff meetings by openly sharing new ideas and information. The flow of ideas is one of the best ways to prevent organizational stagnation.

3) RECOGNIZE ACHIEVEMENT. The supervisor should openly recognize individuals who successfully implement changes and achieve results. Reinforcing the positive aspects of change will allow subordinates to recognize how important change is to the organization.

Resistance to change may also be evidenced in situations where it is obvious that a subordinate is only half listening to what is being said. When confronted with this problem, thoroughly reflect on the manner in which the message was delivered. A subordinate will generally listen to what the supervisor has to say unless it is perceived as irreconcilable or threatening. The manner in which the message is delivered has a significant impact on the impression it leaves with the subordinate.

When assuming a new supervisory position, do not become eager to immediately implement change. A mistake commonly made by those new to health care management is to aggressively assume control and move quickly to solve all the "problems" created by the last supervisor. Give subordinates a period of time, maybe three weeks to two months, to become acquainted with you and your style of leadership. Moving quickly to correct problems may be met with resistance by employees who were comfortable with present operations. Decreases in morale and productivity may result especially if employees helped the previous supervisor implement the present way of doing this. A more satisfactory approach is to announce to all subordinates that some changes are likely to be made but that they will be advised before the changes are introduced. Following this approach lets employees know changes are imminent and reduces the likelihood of resistance.

Avoiding Breakdowns in Communication

Breakdowns in communication can be a common occurrence in a health care organization. The reasons for the breakdowns can often be tied to either the organization itself or to key individuals in management positions. Rarely can the director of the physical therapy department change the entire communications network within an organization. The physical therapist can, however, affect changes within the department which enhance its performance and the level of care offered to the patient. The following provides a number of recommendations for avoiding breakdowns in communication.

1) PREPARE FOR WHAT YOU INTEND TO COMMUNICATE. The imparting of knowledge and information should not be exercised in a haphazard manner. One of the best ways to avoid creating a breakdown in communication is to understand what it is you plan to communicate and select the best method for delivering the message. Only after you have a complete understanding of the material can you be confident of your ability to explain it to subordinates. If your thought process is not clear, chances are the message will be disorganized and difficult to understand by the intended audience.

2) WHO IS THE AUDIENCE? Attempt to learn as much about an audience before you meet with them. Anticipate how they are likely to react to your message and formulate possible answers to the questions that will be asked. Recognize that there are good and bad times to discuss any topic. For example, asking the staff to remain late on Friday afternoon to attend a meeting is likely to be met with formidable opposition. To obtain the best results, always try to structure the timing and content of the message so that it will not be in conflict with the values or beliefs of those it is designed to influence.

3) ALWAYS REQUEST FEEDBACK. One of the most convenient means of ascertaining the comprehension of a managerial communication is to request feedback from the subordinate. Feedback can be obtained in any number of ways. The supervisor can watch for and learn how to interpret non-verbal cues such as an expression of dislike, confusion, a frown, or anger. Another method to use in obtaining feedback is to ask the receiver questions concerning the subject matter. The supervisor may occasionally request the receiver of the message to rephrase its content in his or her own words. If the supervisor does not get the information back in the same manner in which it was communicated, the subordinate should be encouraged to ask questions to obtain further clarification.

MANAGEMENT AND LEARNING HOW TO LISTEN

One of the best ways to avoid developing roadblocks or barriers to communication is for the supervisor to develop the art of becoming a good listener. In patient care, the health care professional who listens to what the patient has to say will learn more about the individual and his or her particular set of needs. The same is true when leading a group of health care professionals. The manager who can take an active interest in employees will learn more about their concerns and about the jobs which they are performing. The only way you can fully convince an employee or a patient of your genuine interest in them is to set aside enough time to fully listen to what they have to say.

This is not to say you must be in complete agreement with what is being said. In many cases you may sharply disagree with the ideas and opinions the subordinate is expressing. The objective of becoming a good listener is to reduce misunderstandings and improve the process of communication in the organization. Additionally, the supervisor who takes an interest in understanding what a subordinate is communicating increases the chances of developing an appropriate response to the questions or comments the individual is attempting to communicate.

Developing proper listening skills is understandably not an easy process. The primary difficulty arises from the fact that the human thought process moves more rapidly than the ability to verbalize. The average person speaks at a rate of approximately 150 words per minute but can listen up to a capacity of 1,000 words per minute. As a result, it is easy to anticipate what someone is going to say or, worse yet, to daydream throughout the conversation. To avoid problems such as this, the supervisor should develop the mental ability to take notes on what is being said and then reduce them into summary form. Attempting to summarize what a subordinate has said will provide a greater opportunity to analyze the true intent of the conversation. In some cases an employee may verbalize or indicate one message when in reality they are attempting to communicate something else. Only through conscious effort can the supervisor develop improved listening skills.

The following are recommended guidelines for increasing the manager's ability to listen.

1) Some health care managers believe that it is part of their responsibility as leaders to carry a majority of a conversation with a subordinate. Nothing could be further from the truth. Those health care managers and leaders who are good listeners stop talking and set aside sufficient time to listen to what is being said.

2) Work to instill confidence in the person who is speaking. Let the individual communicate freely without developing the feeling of being pressured to finish what is being said.

3) Always demonstrate interest in the subordinate's message. Do not allow yourself to be distracted by outside interests which indicate you are not listening to what is being said.

4) Always provide the opportunity for an employee to speak with you in private. When necessary, encourage the employee to discuss the situation in your office away from the daily operations of the department.

5) As supervisor, try to imagine you are in the subordinate's position. Demonstrate empathy and attempt to visualize what the person is going through and how difficult the information may be to discuss.

6) Health care management frequently requires patience. No matter how heated a conversation may become, allow the individual to finish what they are saying. Never walk away in the middle of a conversation.

7) Refrain from any demonstration of anger. The supervisor who loses control of his or her emotions stands a much better chance of verbalizing in an unprofessional manner.

8) Avoid becoming overly critical of any element of subordinate performance. Regardless of the severity of an employee action, avoid criticizing the individual in front of others.

9) Whenever possible, end a conversation on a positive note. This can serve to lessen subordinate anxiety and allow the conversation to be resumed at a later date without residual tension.

10) Show interest in the conversation. Ask questions and make comments which demonstrates an interest in the subject matter.

11) Help the subordinate find a viable solution. If necessary, help in the development of alternative solutions. Encourage the subordinate to select a course of action and strive to create an atmosphere which stimulates goal achievement.

12) Throughout the conversation establish eye contact. Lack of eye contact may leave an impression of disinterest.

FOLLOWING THROUGH WITH ANNOUNCED PLANS

As a health care professional, you have undoubtedly discovered the importance of following through on statements which have been made to patients. When providing health care services, patients respond best to scheduled appointments, consistency in treatment, and a therapist who can be relied upon to do what should be done. The same holds true for health care supervision.

The supervisor who repeatedly fails to follow through on what has been communicated eventually suffers a loss of credibility. Subordinates expect stability and consistency of action from the administration of the organization. This does not fail to recognize the sometimes uncomfortable fact that following through may be personally and professionally difficult for the health care manager. In some instances the price to pay for following through may be so stressful that the supervisor will try to avoid it at all costs.

Regardless of the difficulty of the situation, the health care supervisor is recognized as a vital part of the nucleus of the organization. By choosing to occupy a managerial position the supervisor understands subordinates will listen to and observe what the manager says and does. Some supervisors may, for example, state they maintain an open-door policy in their department. An open-door policy is designed to increase the flow of communication within a department and lessen the opportunity for barriers of communication to develop. Implementing an open-door policy encourages subordinates to come to the supervisor's office, whenever necessary, and discuss personal or organizational problems. A much different message is conveyed when the manager simply remains in the office with the door closed and repeatedly asks not to be disturbed.

MANAGEMENT AND THE NEED TO BE REDUNDANT

Success in health care management often necessitates a message be repeated. In situations where the message is important, complicated, or presents a considerable amount of new or technical language, there is always the chance at least part of the message will be misunderstood. Factors such as the content of the message, and the background and experience of the employee, will further influence the way in which the message is received. Whenever there is evidence of confusion or misunderstanding, being slightly redundant helps ensure the manager is understood.

The process of being redundant must proceed with caution. A message should never be so repetitious that it implies you are talking down to patients, subordinates, or fellow health care professionals. Also, the more familiar the message, the more likely the subordinate is to become disinterested and ignore some of what has been said. For the best results, design your message to stimulate interest and achieve results.

REFERENCES

1. John Fielden, "What Do You Mean I Can't Write?" Harvard Business Review, 42, (May–June 1964), pp. 144–156.
2. D. Katz & R. Kahn, The Social Psychology of Organizations, 2nd ed. (New York: John Wiley & Sons, 1978), p. 440.

Chapter Six

MANAGING GROUPS IN HEALTH CARE ORGANIZATIONS

GROUPS IN HEALTH CARE ORGANIZATIONS
  Formal And Informal Groups
THE FORMATION OF INFORMAL GROUPS
INFORMAL GROUP STRUCTURE
  Group Norms
  Group Roles
  Status Levels
  Group Goals
  Group Member Cohesiveness
ROLE CONFLICT
THE COMMITTEE: A SPECIAL-PURPOSE GROUP
  Types of Committees
  Advantages of Committees and Task Forces
  Disadvantages of Committees and Task Forces
GUIDELINES FOR MAKING GROUPS AND COMMITTEES MORE EFFECTIVE
IMPLICATIONS FOR HEALTH CARE MANAGERS

In the modern health care environment the physical therapist seldom, if ever, acts independently without being influenced by the groups to which he or she belongs. Most physical therapists spend a majority of their health care career working directly with fellow health care professionals, doctors, professional associations, and similar work groups. Each of us behaves differently when associated with a group versus acting on our own.

The purpose of a health care organization is to arrange group activities so members can work effectively toward the common objective of providing quality health care services. The health care organization, whether it be a hospital, nursing home, or private practice physical therapy center, derives its strength from the effective functioning of groups. Understanding group processes is important to the physical therapy supervisor. A thorough understanding of group processes helps ensure the proper management of professionals and non-professionals within the health care organization.

The purpose of this chapter is to introduce the supervisor to the complexities of groups within the formal organization. All health care organizations contain both formal and informal groups. Many factors influence whether an organization blends together in a cohesive manner or operates despite the many role conflicts or cliques which are present. For most health care managers, success will be a direct result of the ability to work effectively with groups. The health care professional must influence the group in order to make effective organizational contributions.

Before reading this chapter, read and answer the following ten questions. Understanding the importance of groups in health care organizations, and using them to your advantage, requires recognizing the varying influences they can have on your ability to supervise them effectively.

Answer true or false:

1) T F Many of the behaviors exhibited by health care professionals and non-professionals are influenced by the groups to which they belong.

2) T F The supervisor's ultimate success depends on his or her ability to work with groups.

3) T F An individual's behavior while in a group will often differ from their behavior outside of the group.

4) T F Leadership ability is enhanced when the supervisor can work effectively with small groups.

5) T F If members of a group place a high value on providing quality patient care, the individual may perform better than if they were not a member of the group.

6) T F There are documented instances where individuals have been suspended or fired from union jobs for working at speeds above the normal standard.

7) T F The individual learns to determine the appropriate behavior in different group situations.

8) T F A group that is experiencing internal conflict is more attractive to members than one where relationships are pleasant and cooperative.

9) T F When an individual group member falls below or exceeds

what is expected by the group, members will exert
pressure to correct the deviation from the norm.

10) T F When a group shares a common fate as a result of an external
attack, such as unjust criticism by a medical doctor or
another health care professional, the group usually becomes more attractive to its members.

Answers: 1, T; 2, T; 3, T; 4, T; 5, T; 6, T; 7, T; 8, F; 9, T; 10, T.

GROUPS IN HEALTH CARE ORGANIZATIONS

Many physical therapists accept their first managerial position expecting
a job requiring considerable time devoted to planning, decision making,
directing and independent thought. Although a considerable period of
time will be spent on each of these functions, a vast majority of the
supervisor's time will be spent directing a group of fellow health care
professionals. For some managers it is not uncommon to spend as much
as 50 percent of their time in one form of group activity or another.

The importance of understanding group processes cannot be over-
emphasized. For purposes of this chapter, a group shall be defined as a
collection of two or more individuals who share a common set of interests,
have frequent interactions, and achieve common objectives and goals.
Understanding these factors is crucial to success in health care management.
Each of these characteristics identify the interdependent relationship the
supervisor has with members of his or her department or practice.

Formal and Informal Groups

A group specifically created by the organization in order to provide an
organized set of health care services and meet established objectives and
goals is referred to as a formal group. Formal groups are present throughout the hospital environment. The departments of physical therapy,
nursing, pediatrics, radiology, and medical records are all examples of
formal groups. The employees in each of these departments share similar tasks and interact with one another to provide patient-related services.

Depending on how well members of a group interact with one another
they may develop beyond just accomplishing their patient care assignments. A group may begin to exhibit activity or behavior which extends
beyond the requirements established by the health care organization.

Members of the group may find others who they would like to interact with or with whom they share a common bond. When this occurs an informal group has developed.

An informal group consists of those individuals with mutual interests, attractions, desires, and needs. Membership in an informal group may or may not include all members of a department. For example, several members from the departments of physical therapy, nursing, and dietary could interact at a social function that is not related to employment at the health care facility. In this case their mutual interests may or may not include subjects related to health care. The primary differences between formal and informal groups can be further examined in Figure 6-1.

FORMAL GROUPS

Created for a specific activity by the organization. Share similar activities, skills, objectives and organizational goals. Membership in the group is required for employment.

INFORMAL GROUPS

Are not created by the health care organization. May not share common tasks or activities. Do share similar values, attitudes and non-organizational goals. Have a membership that is voluntary rather than required.

Figure 6-1.

THE FORMATION OF INFORMAL GROUPS

The creation of the department of physical therapy is a deliberately planned activity on the part of the health care organization. Physical therapists, physical therapy assistants, aides, and supervisors were all acquired by the organization and placed in the department for the purpose of achieving specific objectives and goals. The informal group is not, however, formed with such deliberation. Even though the formation of informal groups is not a planned activity, they do have a rational purpose and share a similar structure. Their purpose and structure are similar to that of the formal group.

A number of factors influence the formation of informal groups. First of all, the supervisor must realize that informal group development is inevitable. Wherever health care organizations exist, people will share common values and attitudes which are considered conducive to group formation. Many health care managers, when asked about groups, immediately discuss what they perceive are the negative aspects of group formation. Those physical therapists who understand the multiple number of reasons why groups form are able to recognize their potential benefits. Once the supervisor understands informal group development, he or she can then influence the group and encourage members to make very positive organizational contributions.

One of the primary reasons why informal groups develop is because of proximity. This is easy to understand, since most of our daily employment interactions are with those individuals who work with us in the same department. Relationships and friendships commonly develop in the working environment because the physical proximity makes these relationships possible. We often work with the same group of people eight to ten hours per day. It is only natural to share similar interests and develop friendships with those who assist us in providing health care services.

Group membership also provides the individual with an opportunity to engage in a number of professional and non-professional interactions. These interactions include working with individuals who have differing levels of professional background and experience. Due to the extensive communication network that is established in most health care organizations, the health care professional will have the opportunity to interact with fellow health care professionals, doctors, nurses, and clerical personnel. Although much of the communication will concern professional matters, ample opportunity exists to share information which has little or nothing to do with providing health care services.

Interpersonal attraction is another factor that influences the emergence of an informal group. When group members share similar attitudes, values, and personality characteristics there is a greater chance an informal group will develop. People may also be attracted to one another because of similar beliefs or like economic situations. Interestingly enough, employees who share similar characteristics are more likely to form an informal group than employees who do not share similarities but interact more frequently.

Employees are also likely to form informal groups in reaction to anxiety, pleasure, frustration, or similar emotions about their jobs. Employees often share emotional reactions to jobs which extend from very pleasurable to unpleasurable to somewhere in between. In many instances groups form to allow employees to share emotion and reduce tension concerning a certain aspect of their job. An informal group that develops as a result of unpleasant feelings about a job allows members to openly express their dissatisfaction with others who have similar reactions to the demands of the job.

INFORMAL GROUP STRUCTURE

When examining informal group structure within a health care organization it becomes readily apparent that group members have a number of similarities as well as differences. Even though members share common beliefs, values, and attitudes there may still be differences in opinion as to how to proceed in solving a particular problem. Some employees will outwardly verbalize their feelings about a problem, while others will carefully examine the situation from a distance and without comment. It is not uncommon for some employees to attempt to "take charge," while others prefer to be less influential. How a group is structured provides the means by which members regulate their behavior.

Group structure is the consistent relationships among members as those relationships become established and implicitly accepted by the members.[1] Within each group there is a structure similar to that of the formal organization. There are leaders, followers, goals, and accepted behaviors. In the formal group there are written rules of conduct and specified working relationships. The informal group rarely has written codes of conduct, yet each member of the group is generally aware of the groups structure and working relationships and can frequently verbalize it.

A number of factors influence the relationship among group members. The six most common influencing factors are: group norms, group roles, status levels, group goals, group member cohesiveness and role conflict.

Group Norms

Group norms are values and rules of conduct members have established to maintain desired group behavior. Norms represent ideal group member behavior. Members of a health care management team in an organization may establish norms, but they must be accepted by the various groups within the organization if they are to become worthwhile and meaningful. Norms are, as such, situational. They apply only to situations that are important to the group but do not cover all behaviors in every possible situation. Violation of established norms carries with it penalties such as ridicule, embarrassment, or loss of group membership.

Groups most often develop norms which they find to be useful in directing the behavior of others. Norms may become very powerful in standardizing the things you should do, the things you should not do, and the things that are considered acceptable. Health care professionals and non-professionals may violate norms but will quickly be subjected to group pressure to correct the deviation from acceptable behavior. This will be especially true if the behavior continues for a long period of time.

An example of a "should not" norm includes, you should not criticize the behavior or treatment methods of another health care professional in front of a patient. Examples of a "should" norm includes, as department director you should attend the hospital's Christmas party. An example of a "may" norm includes, as supervisor you may encourage a subordinate to come speak with you about personal problems or concerns, but the organization does not require it.

In most instances, norms will be broad, specifying a wide range of acceptable behaviors. They seldom specify just one way an individual may behave. The less important the issue, the wider the range of acceptable behavior. Norms which involve the achievement of a major group goal, its continued existence, or threaten the identity or reputation of the group carry a much narrower range of acceptable behaviors.

For the health care manager it is important to recognize group norms and support those activities that contribute toward achieving organizational objectives and goals. The manager should never discourage group formation but instead follow the development of the group and work to influence norms in a positive manner. The norms established by a group can profoundly influence productivity within the organization. At all levels the worker is influenced by group norms and pressured to conform. If the manager recognizes that certain group norms lead to increased productivity, considerable benefit can be derived from encouraging strong group loyalties.

Group Roles

A group role refers to the expectations shared by group members regarding who does which task and under what conditions.[2] In a formal health care setting, such as in the department of physical therapy, behavioral expectations are defined by use of the job description. In contrast, the informal role expectations are never recorded in writing but instead are developed by group members as a result of job experience.

Within the physical therapy department there are many tasks to be performed, only part of which are determined by the supervisor. Other functions performed by the worker are considered informal and serve social functions. All members of a health care organization develop an understanding as to the activities they should and should not perform. Each health care professional will define the roles that other members of a group should assume or not assume. These roles are based on individual perceptions, beliefs, attitudes, and feelings about what is correct and incorrect in the working environment. Within each group, members will take on both informal and formal roles. For example, one staff therapist may specialize in certain formal work roles, perhaps serving as an expert on rehabilitation of total knee replacements. Other therapists may specialize in the informal social roles such as planning group activities and making the organization a stimulating place to work.

Status Levels

Status is the position or rank an individual holds in a group.[3] To coordinate social and work activities the behavior of each member must be adjusted to that of the others. Status recognizes that a person's rank is based upon the needs of group members while at the same time accomplishing group objectives and goals.

Within the modern health care organization two forms of status can be identified: formal and informal status. Formal status is the position or rank the person holds within the health care organization. Examples include chief executive officer, director of rehabilitative services, and assistant director of physical therapy. Each of these positions recognizes status as designated by the organization.

Informal status is the social standing the individual has received by the evaluation of the group. Within the department there may be one or more group members who do not hold a management position but are recognized as leaders. These are individuals who can generally offer sound advice or guidance on group-related matters.

Both types of status have a profound influence on how individuals behave in health care organizations. Those physical therapists who have charisma and occupy management positions can attract other professionals to the organization. Some professionals consider status as a factor which must be evaluated when considering joining a group or organization. High-status groups will often attract more members than low-status groups. Health care professionals with high-status needs may accept jobs with low pay, at least for awhile, to fulfill these needs. To some, achieving status is more important than the amount of pay that is provided. A manager should attempt to identify those professionals who seek status and are effective at motivating a group. For the health care supervisor, proper identification of those individuals who have the important social and task-related skills is important. Individuals respected by a group can be of assistance to the manager in gaining the group's support for organizational objectives and goals.

Group Goals

Informal groups often emerge because of some purpose to which the members are committed. A union may form as a result of worker dissatisfaction and a strong desire to change the organization and its working conditions. A goal gives the group a reason to exist and to continue forward. Depending on the goal selected, it can have dramatic effects on group behavior. Some hospitals, for example, have been unionized due to employee dissatisfaction. Members join the union to hopefully force changes in their working conditions and improve their individual economic situations. Here, the group goal is clear: to make the hospital a better place to work.

Group Member Cohesiveness

Group member cohesiveness refers to the amount of attraction group members have to one another and the degree to which they are committed to moving in the same direction. The cohesiveness of the group affects its stability. Cohesiveness reinforces group roles, goals, norms, status levels, and is directly related to group member satisfaction. Those workers who are members of cohesive groups often work harder to achieve group goals than those who belong to less cohesive groups. Members of highly cohesive groups are also less likely to be absent from work.

A number of factors influence the degree to which a group becomes cohesive. The primary influencing factors are: group size, the effect of working on common goals, the ability of the group leader to facilitate cohesion, loyalty to the group, responsibility for group activities, identification with the group, agreement with group goals, conformity to group norms, and acceptance of group decisions. Their effect on group cohesiveness is demonstrated in Figure 6-2.

As a physical therapy supervisor your primary concern with a group's cohesiveness is that the group adopts goals which are similar to organizational goals. If group goals and organizational goals are similar, the cohesiveness is positive for the health care facility. It is the similarity between adopted goals and formal goals that directly affects productivity.[4]

In a health care organization a number of factors can influence the degree to which membership in a group is attractive. The following is an outline for increasing group cohesiveness and for avoiding those factors which decrease group productivity.

Factors Increasing Group Cohesiveness

1) The more status a group receives, the more attractive to potential members.
2) When attacked from an outside source, a group usually becomes more cohesive.
3) When there is little or no internal competition, group cohesiveness is higher.
4) The more prestige group members receive, the more attractive group membership becomes.

Factors Decreasing Group Cohesiveness

1) The greater the level of interpersonal conflict, the less attractive group membership will be.
2) If membership in a group results in the members being embarrassed, the attractiveness of the group will decrease.
3) When membership in the group becomes confining or limits the

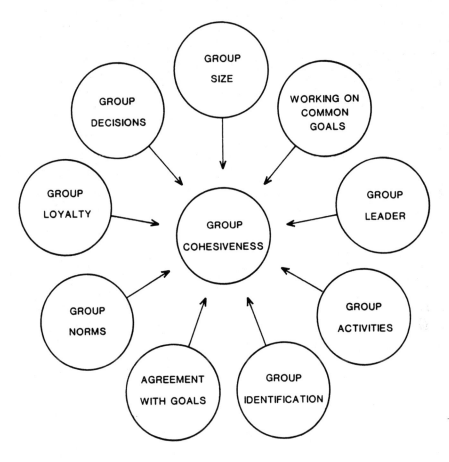

Figure 6-2.

individual's participation in other groups or activities, the attractiveness of the group will be lessened.

4) If conditions are present in the group which limit members from satisfying social needs, such as for belonging or friendship, the level of cohesiveness will be reduced.

5) If members of the group perceive adverse personal or professional risks associated with group membership or engaging in its activities, attractiveness will be decreased.

6) If the group receives negative feedback from an outsider whose opinions and ideas are valued and respected, group cohesiveness may be lowered.

In general, the attractiveness of the group will increase the more it satisfies members' needs for recognition and achievement. When members can communicate freely and engage in pleasant interpersonal relationships, cohesiveness will be increased. If the individual determines that participation in the group no longer meets his or her needs or they can better be satisfied elsewhere, membership will no longer appear as rewarding.

The results of increased cohesiveness can have a very positive influence on a health care organization. A department of physical therapy which has a number of highly cohesive groups is quite often aware of its strengths and its limitations. The organization and its members are cognizant of how much each member should contribute to group productivity. When a group member does not conform to what is expected, pressure will be applied to bring the person "into line." Productivity will also be adjusted so that it conforms with group norms. If the group strongly agrees with the objectives and goals established by management, achievement will be markedly higher than if the group objects to what has been proposed. The physical therapy supervisor must, therefore, recognize the degree of group cohesiveness and work with, not against, developing a productive relationship.

ROLE CONFLICT

For the physical therapist, role conflict occurs whenever the individual is faced with role expectations that are incompatible with what he or she believes is inherently correct. For example, if role expectations of a small community hospital are that all physician orders must be followed explicitly, whereas the therapist's role expectations are that some orders are not in the patients best interest, a role conflict may result. The therapist may experience personal conflict from trying to balance the two sets of expectations.

Role conflict can have its origin in any number of professional and non-professional forces but will occur more frequently in situations where role expectations are rigidly enforced by a group. The effect the conflict has on the individual depends on his or her ability to ignore conflicting role expectations.

Presently, the profession of physical therapy is, as a whole, strongly against the employment of physical therapists in physician-owned facilities. Some members of the profession have taken very strong positions on the matter and have gone as far as accusing those members of the profession who work in such facilities as "selling out the profession." For the physical therapist employed in a physician-owned facility, role conflict may result if the therapist trys to balance continued loyalty to the profession and retain employment at the facility.

THE COMMITTEE: A SPECIAL-PURPOSE GROUP

Almost every hospital, rehabilitation center, nursing home or medium-sized business has a committee. A committee is a special-purpose group usually characterized by a designated membership, a chairperson, secretary, and with somewhat regular meetings. Committees, especially in large health care organizations, are a major part of the organization's structure. To some, membership on a committee is an honor or a symbol of status. Still others consider it time consuming and do their best to avoid becoming a member.

Committees can serve a number of very important purposes. Some of the most frequently identified are:[5]

1) To provide managers with an opportunity to exchange information and differing views on a variety of subjects.
2) To generate ideas or solutions to organizational problems.
3) To make recommendations to higher level management.
4) To actually make decisions.

In health care, committees also provide a number of additional functions. They include:

1) To coordinate the efforts of a large number of specialized professional and non-professional people.
2) To develop treatment programs which enhance the organization's prestige in the community, state, or nation.
3) To improve communication between medical doctors, the administration, and hospital personnel.
4) To develop and coordinate fund-raising activities for the expansion of the facility.

Due to the increasing complexity and rate of change in health care organizations today, the committee serves as one of the best ways of pooling the expertise of different members of an organization. It also provides an opportunity for channeling the efforts of a large number of highly skilled professionals toward effective problem solving and decision making.

Types Of Committees

Large health care organizations, such as major medical centers, often have a number of committees which differ regarding their purpose, decision-making authority, frequency of meetings, and membership. Three types of committees can be identified.

1) TASK FORCE. A task force, sometimes referred to as a project team, is formed to deal with a specific issue, task, problem, or purpose. The group is in existence only until the problem or purpose is completed after which the individual members return to their normal duties. A task force will generally consist of key people from several departments within the hospital. A task force may, for example, be created from members of the departments of medical records, outpatient billing, physical therapy, and occupational therapy. Their purpose may be to coordinate the billing, scheduling, and record keeping of patients who are to be seen on an outpatient basis.

2) PERMANENT OR STANDING COMMITTEES. Permanent or standing committees are established to meet a continuing need or issue within the health care organization. Examples of a standing committee include the curriculum development committee in the department of physical therapy of a university. Here, members will meet on a regular basis to discuss the current educational program and recommend the appropriate changes to present course offerings. One of the primary differences between a task force and a permanent or standing committee is that the committee is generally longer lasting and has a much more stable membership. Members of committees are often chosen because of their titles or positions, whereas task force members are selected because of a skill or expertise and an ability to carry out the given task or assignment.

3) BOARDS. A board is comprised of a specialized group of individuals who have been given the responsibility of managing the health care organization. The members of the board are either appointed or elected for a specified term. Among their numerous responsibilities will include making key decisions concerning the direction and future of the organization. Examples of the decisions made by the board members include issues involving the expansion of the present facility or expanding the services it has to offer.

Advantages of Committees and Task Forces

Health care institutions provide an opportunity to work with people who come from diverse backgrounds with varying levels of training and experience. Committees and task forces are frequently composed of those individuals who have substantial experience and knowledge and can potentially develop more solutions to a problem than could be developed by one person acting alone. Committees offer a number of the following advantages to a health care organization.

1) A committee will often generate better quality decisions than the same number of people working individually on a problem. Members of the group are also more likely to be committed to the final solution, since it was based on group decision making and group consensus. The final solution arrived at by the committee should be the best choice among all of the alternatives developed and discussed.

2) The members of the group often have a proprietary (ownership) feeling about the decision and will take an active interest in its implementation. All members of the committee may not agree with the solution or decision, but at least they will understand the reasoning behind it.

3) Committee decisions help prevent the abuse of power. When a decision is placed in the hands of one person there is an opportunity to abuse power, demonstrate favoritism, make inappropriate decisions, or evidence bias. When responsibility for decision making is evenly distributed among members of a board or committee, it reduces the chances of excessive power being exercised by one individual. Additionally, there are likely to be fewer complaints about a poor decision if several people were responsible for selecting it.

4) Committee membership can be a training ground for future managers, especially for the physical therapist aspiring for a top level management position. Committee involvement can be an excellent way of obtaining experience concerning how top management perceives and deals with problems. The manager can learn how to look at the organization from a conceptual point of view rather than solely focusing on his or her department. The committee also provides an opportunity to evaluate the successful and unsuccessful leadership styles of fellow health care managers.

Disadvantages of Committees and Task Forces

Committees and task forces may also provide a number of disadvantages to the health care organization. The following are some of the most common problems:

1) In some committees or groups, social pressure may serve to intimidate members into accepting a decision which would otherwise be unacceptable. Those committee members who see a solution as personally best for them may strongly encourage others to adopt their same position on the problem.

2) One person may try to assume a leadership role and dominate the group. Sometimes, a strong-willed individual can force acceptance of an unpopular decision. This can be detrimental to the organization if the dominant person is not the best problem solver in the group. Individual domination is not uncommon and, if escalated, may result in a power struggle. People who see themselves as leaders may use the committee to help satisfy their needs to exercise control, power, or dominance.

3) Committee and task force membership can be very time consuming. The time the manager spends on a committee is time which cannot be spent working on the functions for which he or she is payed for. Most committee members strongly resent being a member of a group that is not productive or accomplishes little of what it was organized for.

4) Committee members are generally not accountable for their decisions. It is not uncommon for a committee or task force to make a decision that would have not been made if an individual had to assume full responsibility. As a whole, a group will make a riskier decision than would an individual. Groups can be more bold and daring, since no one member feels solely responsible for the ultimate decision and eventual outcome.

GUIDELINES FOR MAKING
GROUPS AND COMMITTEES MORE EFFECTIVE

Health care professionals, and the committees to which they belong, exert a powerful influence on the management of the institution. The leader of the group or committee must exercise the necessary skills and abilities to encourage followers to complete assigned tasks and act with commitment towards the health care organization's objectives and goals. It is important to recognize the proper steps to take in organizing and directing committees so as to achieve the maximum amount of organizational effectiveness. The following will be of benefit to committee formation in a health care organization.

1) THE PURPOSE OF THE COMMITTEE SHOULD BE CLEARLY DEFINED. All members should have a good understanding of the proposed goals, how much authority they have to gather information, and how soon a decision or recommendation is expected. It is advisable for the committee chairperson to communicate at least some of the basic information to each member in writing prior to the first scheduled meeting. This provides committee members with an opportunity to review the subject matter in advance and prevents unnecessary time devoted to outlining the ultimate objectives and goals of the committee.

2) SELECT THE RIGHT PEOPLE FOR THE COMMITTEE. Proper selection of committee members is essential to ensuring the best decisions and recommendations are developed. It is advantageous to have several experts on the committee who are aware of the problem or issue but have not committed themselves as to what would be the best course of action. In selecting members, try to maintain committee size to between five and ten individuals. The larger the committee, the more time consuming and difficult it will be to manage.

3) DEVELOP AN AGENDA FOR EACH COMMITTEE MEETING. The chairperson of the committee must never arrive at a meeting unprepared. Each member should be provided with an outline of proposed topics for discussion. At the close of each meeting there should be a summation of what has been discussed, as well as proposed topics for the next meeting. Only by keeping the committee focused can the chairperson ensure success.

4) ENCOURAGE MEMBER PARTICIPATION. Whenever groups of professionals are organized together for some specific function there are always individuals who dominate the discussion while others remain silent. When someone is not actively involved in expressing their ideas or opinions, it is the chairperson's responsibility to encourage participation by asking for input. In situations where group members know little about one another, the chairperson should conduct an informal introduction to help "break the ice."

5) Keep the Meetings Moving. The chairperson should set a time limit for each meeting and follow the agenda. The longer the meeting lasts, the more likely group members are to become distracted. Knowing what subjects are to be covered and how much time will be devoted to each will help keep the direction of the committee focused.

IMPLICATIONS FOR HEALTH CARE MANAGERS

The quality of leadership demonstrated by the health care supervisor is one of the most important ingredients for ensuring success in group management. Additionally, the physical therapist must recognize the influence that norms, status, and role conflict have on group cohesion and commitment toward organizational objectives and goals. The objectives and goals of the organization can only be attained through the effective coordination of groups.

Groups provide a number of important functions in a health care organization. Beyond just providing patient care, groups help to satisfy the needs of both professional and non-professional personnel. Since much of a physical therapy supervisor's job involves activities such as leading, it is important to understand which factors influence group performance.

Group norms and cohesiveness are two of the most powerful factors in determining group performance. A group where members conform to established norms and are highly cohesive will have a positive influence on performance. In order to be effective, the health care manager must understand what the groups norms are and how they operate within the organization. The manager should also attempt to identify the informal group leader and develop a positive working relationship with that individual.

The supervisor of physical therapy must endeavor to support positive group efforts and outwardly recognize the contributions the group makes to the health care organization. Only when the manager recognizes how a group contributes to the success or failure of the department will the individual devote sufficient attention to effective management of group processes.

REFERENCES

1. D. Cartwright and A. Zander, Group Dynamics (New York: Harper & Row, 1968), p. 486.
2. L. Porter, E. Lawler, III, & J. Hackman, Behavior in Organizations (New York: McGraw-Hill, 1975), p. 373.
3. Cartwright, op., cit., p. 215.
4. B. L. Hinton, & H. J. Reitz, Groups and Organizations (Belmont, CA: Wadsworth, 1971), p. 126.
5. "Committees: Their Role in Management Today," Management Review (October 1957), pp. 4–10.

Chapter Seven

STRESS AND HEALTH CARE MANAGEMENT

It is understandable that most health care organizations place a high value on those physical therapists who assume managerial positions. The supervisor of a department is responsible for providing the necessary direction, motivation, leadership, and control that ensures workers perform their jobs and patients receive quality care. An understanding of job-related stress is important to managers. Prolonged stress can have serious physical and psychological side effects on health care professionals. Some studies indicate the side effects of stress are particularly pronounced in managerial personnel.

Stress is increasingly more common in the health care environment. Today's health care professional is under more and more time constraints to provide quality care in shorter periods of time. Patients, family members, private insurance companies, and the federal government all bear the burden of paying for the rising costs of health care. Increasingly, the burden is being shifted to medical doctors and to the rehabilitation specialists to correct a patient's physical disorder with a cost-efficient delivery of health care services.

Stress can be a major cause of employee turnover and absenteeism. As the director of a physical therapy department the individual is continually caught between trying to meet the needs of subordinates while at the same time trying to ensure the department meets the needs of the organization and the patients it serves. Every health care manager experiences stress trying to cope with the day-to-day problems presented in a department. How the professional handles stress is an important aspect of health care supervision. Some estimates indicate that between 80 and 90 percent of industrial accidents are caused by personal factors.[1] The more the manager knows about stress and its effects, the less likely it will be manifested as counterproductive behavior.

Stress may indeed produce undesirable effects on the health care supervisor. At low levels, stress may only produce such symptoms as indigestion, fatigue, and mild headache. As the level of stress increases it can have undesirable side effects such as ulcers, high blood pressure and stroke. How much stress a person can handle depends on the type of stress and the ability of the person to handle a pressure situation. Stress at moderate levels can result in higher performance and be recognized as a positive force. Understanding what stress is and how to adapt to it is crucial to your effectiveness in health care management.

THE NATURE OF STRESS

Stress is a consequence of or a response to an action, situation, or force that places special physical demands, psychological demands, or both, on a person.[2] Stress specifically involves the interactions of a person with situations presented in an environment. Every health care professional has experienced the feelings that result from stress. They include tension, rapid speech, racing heart, perspiration, and a dry mouth. Stress is a normal reaction to conflict or frustration as the individual attempts to adapt to the pressures of a job. Stress is not something which can be avoided when occupying a managerial position. In fact, it may be increased significantly as the physical therapist assumes increasing responsibilities.

The physiological reactions of increased pulse, rapid uptake of oxygen, elevated blood pressure, pupil dilation, and increased muscle tension occur to at least some degree each time the individual prepares to meet a challenge. Some managers react differently to stress than others. An individual may find one situation as producing high levels of anxiety while others find the same situation a major source of satisfaction. It is important to keep in mind that stress for one person may be quite desirable for another. People react differently to stress and vary in how much stress can effectively be handled.

SOME CAUSES OF STRESS

There are a large number of factors which are recognized as having the potential for inducing anxiety in both managerial and non-managerial personnel. A number of studies have been conducted which have identified specific stressors and their effects.[3] Although work stressors can take on a variety of forms, there are a few common causes. Figure 7-1 depicts some of the most common causes.

Organizational Change

For a supervisor, stress will be perceived in each instance where the organization requires the implementation of a new policy, procedure, or method of operation which is opposed to how it has been done in the past. If the supervisor perceives a new responsibility as stressful because of the changes which are required, it may be anxiety producing. In situations such as this, the stress perceived by the supervisor will result

```
┌─────────────────────────────────────────────┐
│                                               │
│              SOURCES OF STRESS                │
│         ──────────────────────────           │
│                                               │
│            Organizational Change             │
│                                               │
│            Individual Personality            │
│                                               │
│               Role Ambiguity                 │
│                                               │
│                Role Conflict                 │
│                                               │
│          Lack of Management Support          │
│                                               │
│          Middle Management Positions         │
│                                               │
│   Relationships with Subordinates and Colleagues │
│                                               │
│          Physical Working Conditions         │
│                                               │
│        Quantitative / Qualitative Overload   │
│                                               │
│        Quantitative / Qualitative Underload  │
│                                               │
│                Time Pressures                │
│                                               │
│             Lack of Participation            │
│                                               │
│              Poor Communications             │
│                                               │
└─────────────────────────────────────────────┘
```

Figure 7-1.

from having to convince subordinates of its importance. If, for example, the hospital's chief administrator wants physical therapy provided seven days a week when it has not been provided in that manner before, the responsibility for recruiting weekend workers may be quite stressful on the manager.

Individual Personality

As is well known, cardiovascular disease is one of the leading causes of death in the United States. More than 40 million people are afflicted with some form of heart disease. Approximately one million will die each year.[4]

Meyer Friedman and Ray Rosenman are two medical cardiologists and researchers who, in the 1950s, discovered what they termed were "Type A" and Type B" behavior patterns.[5] As a result of their extensive research, it was determined that the traditional risk factors such as dietary cholesterol, high blood pressure, and the person's heredity could not, by themselves, fully be used to predict heart disease. Through the process of interviewing and observing specific patient behavior they uncovered behaviors which they believe are related to coronary heart disease. Individuals with a "Type A" behavior pattern demonstrate the following characteristics:

- They are always in a hurry to get as many things done as possible in the shortest period of time.
- They can be characterized as impatient. The individual dislikes waiting and considers waiting a waste of valuable time.
- They often speak rapidly and are known to interrupt others in the course of a conversation.
- They may be characterized as work oriented and preoccupied with deadlines.
- They may be aggressive, ambitious, and competitive.
- They may repeatedly be in a struggle with people, things, and events.

In comparison to the "Type A" behavior pattern, the person classified as "Type B" presents a more confident style that allows work to be performed at a steady pace and not against the clock. The "Type B" personality seldom desires to accomplish increasingly large numbers of objectives or to participate in more activities. The "Type B" personality has the opposite characteristics of the "Type A" individual.[6] The "Type B" may possess considerable drive and will work hard but will be less likely to overreact to situations, less likely to be competitive, less status conscious, and insist less on recognition for achievement than the "Type A" individual. Some of those work events or situations that are bothersome to "Type A" individuals may be considered unimportant to "Type B" individuals. People with "Type B" characteristics often feel there is sufficient time to get things done. This does not imply, however, that they lack desire for career success or goal accomplishment.

In describing the "Type A" behavior pattern, the researchers examined the results of wear on the chairs in their office waiting room. An upholsterer had been called to make repairs on a number of chairs that evidenced wear. When the upholsterer inspected the chairs, he questioned as to what speciality of medicine the physicians were practicing. The upholsterer had noticed that the front edge of each chair was worn. The cardiologist's interpreted this finding to mean that some of the patients were sitting on the edge of their chairs waiting impatiently to be seen. "Type A" individuals, who are naturally somewhat impatient with waiting, would tend to evidence such behavior.

Role Ambiguity

When an individual experiences role ambiguity they believe they lack clear job objectives. A supervisor who lacks a full understanding of what performance is expected will experience stress. Those physical therapists new to a supervisory position may experience role ambiguity until they become familiar with the responsibilities and demands of the job. Every new job will present certain levels of role ambiguity in the first few weeks. If the ambiguity extends beyond two to three weeks, the individual will begin to recognize it as a source of stress.

Role Conflict

The supervisor or staff physical therapist who is experiencing role conflict feels as though the stress is the result of conflicting job demands or expectations. To perform a job faster, cut corners, or even to improve performance may not be possible when delivering health care services. The supervisor may, for example, want each physical therapist to treat more patients. The consequence may be a reduction in the quality of care the patient receives. Requiring more patients to be treated and witnessing a declining quality of care may be stressful to the supervisor and to the subordinates. Role conflict is often experienced by supervisors when the job requires an increasing number of hours be devoted while family members require additional attention.

Lack of Management Support

A supervisor who lacks the support and backing of top management may have increased difficulty in performing a job. The supervisor may, for example, recognize the need to expand the number of staff physical therapists. If top management repeatedly fails to respond to requests for additional staff, the manager may be perceived by subordinates as one who lacks the "clout" to get things done.

Middle Management Positions

Those physical therapists who are directors of departments are frequently in positions of first or middle level management. In most instances they are directly responsible to employees below and to supervisors above. Being in situations where there is an opportunity to be pulled in two directions is stressful. Middle management positions are recognized as some of the most stressful supervisory positions in health care.

Relationships with Subordinates and Colleagues

The director of a physical therapy department will be in contact with a diverse group of people who have varying degrees of background and experience. Interacting with employees can be a particularly stressful experience. Employees may assume the supervisor attained his or her position because of a unique ability to provide answers to questions in a moment's notice. The demands placed on a supervisor by subordinates and colleagues undoubtedly add stress to managerial positions.

Inability to Delegate

Those health care supervisors who try to do it all will soon recognize that most things will only partially get done. In order to be effective in health care management, the supervisor must delegate tasks to others. No supervisor can perform all the tasks required for department operation. In delegating tasks the supervisor must delegate the authority and responsibility to see that the job gets done. Authority is the right to perform a task assigned by the administration of an organization. Responsibility is the right to see that the task is carried out. In order to be effective, the supervisor must delegate both authority and responsibility to the subordinate.

Physical Working Conditions

A physical therapy department that is too noisy, cold, crowded, presents unsafe working conditions, or is uncomfortable will increase the potential for stress. When contemplating a position as director or as a staff therapist, the department must be carefully evaluated. A department which is rundown, understaffed, or has old or inoperable equipment will require the support of top management in order to be corrected. A department which does not have a private office for the director often elevates stress levels when the manager is forced to hunt for a place to discuss personal matters with subordinates.

Quantitative/Qualitative Overload

In the health care environment there are two types of work overload which may be encountered. The first, and most common, is that of quantitative overload. In quantitative overload the person feels as though there is not enough time to properly complete all tasks which are assigned. The director may, for example, be expected to carry the patient load of a staff therapist while at the same time continuing to perform administrative duties. Here, the supervisor develops the feeling of being overwhelmed, which may rapidly lead to job dissatisfaction.

In qualitative overload the supervisor feels as though he or she lacks the experience or abilities to handle a job. Qualitative overload stress is a common complaint of those physical therapists new to health care management. Having just assumed the responsibility for the welfare of subordinates, the new director may look at the job as overwhelming. If the new health care manager resists the urge to panic, the job will become less ominous after about a month. Any new job, especially one that is administrative in nature, requires a period of individual adjustment.

Quantitative/Qualitative Underload

Although it may be quite obvious that the director of physical therapy who is too busy may feel stressed, it is also quite possible that too little work can produce stress. In the situation of quantitative underload a director may have too few administrative tasks to occupy a full day. On a periodic basis this is considered normal, but if it extends to the long term it can be stressful. Individuals placed in positions such as these will attempt to alleviate the feelings of stress by creating "busy work." Trying to look busy will only temporarily relieve the stress associated with long periods of inactivity.

When a supervisor or staff physical therapist experiences qualitative underload it is because the job does not require enough of his or her abilities. As a result, the person will experience boredom which, if allowed to continue, will become stressful. This is the primary reason why many health care organizations look for supervisors who have had careers that demonstrate progressive administrative responsibility. A supervisor who has managed departments with as many as 35 employees may not be sufficiently stimulated by accepting a managerial position in a department with 10 employees. The supervisor must be challenged by the organization or the individual risks the chance of developing apathy.

Time Pressures

Those jobs which present a demanding pace are recognized as being stressful. Individual makeup does play a role, but in general most health care professionals resent being forced to hurry through a day's work. Stress levels will be even higher in departments where the supervisor has little or no sympathy for the pace of the required work.

Lack of Participation

Health care supervisors who feel as though they have little influence concerning the decisions affecting their department are more likely to experience symptoms of stress. When top management makes a majority of the decisions without consulting the supervisor, it leaves the individual with the impression that they are little more than a figurehead. The supervisor will often develop the feeling that they are of insignificant value to the organization. When evaluating the acceptance of a supervisory position it is important to meet and converse with the person to whom you will report. After talking with that person you will immediately know whether you will be expected to follow orders or allowed to be creative. The more participative in decision making your supervisor is, the more likely you are to derive satisfaction from the job.

Poor Communication

The director of physical therapy is primarily responsible for establishing a connecting link between subordinates and the next level of supervision. Poor communication with either party will greatly enhance stress for the supervisor. If the department director cannot openly discuss important topics with the supervisor, the director will soon become frustrated. If, on the other hand, the director does not meet regularly with and communicate to subordinates, they will develop the feeling of alienation. As such, the director of physical therapy is the "one in the middle." Communications must be good above and below if the director is to be effective.

THE CONSEQUENCES OF PROLONGED STRESS

Stress has been reported as a contributing factor in a number of health-related disorders. Although individual ability to cope with stress will vary greatly, there are a number of surprisingly common signs and symptoms. Being able to recognize stressors at work will allow the health care manager to take steps to alleviate many of the most common causes. The five most dangerous and disruptive effects of stress were identified by T. Cox.[7] The categories include:

Organizational

The behaviors of individuals experiencing stress in an organization include increased absenteeism, lower productivity, interpersonal conflict, accidents, turnover, job dissatisfaction, reduced organizational loyalty, and antagonism at work.

Physiological

The most commonly reported individual reactions to stress include: heart attacks, strokes, fatigue, ulcers, increased blood pressure, dryness of the mouth, dilation of the pupils, hot and cold flashes, skin disorders, indigestion, and headaches.

Cognitive Effects

The individual may suffer a loss of concentration, make poor decisions, have a reduced attention span, strongly resist criticism, experience anxiety, depression, aggression or guilt, boredom, feelings of inadequacy, or suffer a low self-esteem.

Behavioral

The behavioral effects of stress are often evidenced through such behaviors as drug abuse, alcoholism, overeating or undereating, the development of nervous gestures, emotional outbursts, changes in sleeping patterns or sleeping too much, a deterioration of interpersonal relationships, impulsive behavior, or nervous laughter.

Subjective Effects

The subjective effects may include the repeated loss of temper or a persistent feeling of being alone. Stress-related illnesses and problems place a considerable burden on the individual and on the health care organization. Clearly, some of the reactions to stress are more obvious on the individual than they are to the organization. Computing the exact costs to an organization is not possible. It is important, however, to be aware of some of the estimated costs associated with increased employee absenteeism, alcoholism, and drug abuse. The effects of these problems can be very costly in terms of organizational productivity.

Absenteeism and Withdrawal

Health care employees who hold positions as managers or non-managers may react to high levels of stress by repeatedly being absent from the job or by leaving it entirely. J.D. Kearns conducted a study over a 15-year period measuring the effects stress on job absenteeism and turnover.[8] The results indicate there was a 22 percent increase in absenteeism directly attributed to physical health problems. Absenteeism, which could be associated with psychological health problems, demonstrated a 152 percent increase for men and 302 percent increase for women.

In another study of 175 hospital employees the researcher was unable to predict turnover but did determine that high levels of stress were significant predictors of an individual's intentions to leave the hospital. It was determined that those employees with low reported stress levels had greater expectations of remaining at the hospital longer.[9]

Alcoholism

The problems with alcoholism and stress have been linked to all levels in the organizational hierarchy. Alcohol may be used by employees to escape from the rigors of a routine or stressful job. Problem drinkers may account for as much as $20 billion each year in sick pay, absenteeism, lost productivity, and the mishandling of resources. It has been estimated that 9 percent of males and 5 percent of females in the United States are at risk for developing alcoholism or a serious drinking problem.[10] No single study has established a firm link between the types of work performed and the use of alcohol as a response to stress. It has been determined that alcoholics have higher needs for emotional support, may be more aggressive, and may be more impulsive when making easy decisions.[11]

One requirement of health care management is to offer to assist those employees who demonstrate an alcohol problem. Unfortunately, the evidence of an alcohol abuse problem is not always clear. In the early stages of the disease the ability to work may show little or no deterioration. As the disease becomes more of a problem, both job quantity and quality will generally suffer.[12]

The treatment for alcoholism tends to be more effective if the disease is identified in its early stages. Although treatment is more effective in the early stages, it may be during that period when the employee is most likely to resist treatment. Instead of firing an employee with an alcohol problem, many experts believe it is better to create a confrontation that leads to the alcoholic admitting there is a problem. Helping to identify a problem requires the manager to be aware of some of the signs and symptoms. Some of the most common are:

- A recognizable pattern of absenteeism is evidenced. The employee will frequently be absent on Mondays and Fridays. The employee will also typically be absent before and after holidays.
- Absences from work increase and they are often unexcused.
- The employee frequently arrives late, may take long lunch breaks, and often desires to leave work early.
- The employee increasingly makes poor decisions and exercises poor judgment.
- Physical appearance begins to deteriorate, the individual may suffer a rapid weight loss, be unclean or unshaven.

- The employee may be more accident prone and have an increase in the number of hospital medical claims.
- The smell of alcohol may be present on the breath or clothing of the individual.
- Job-related performance may decrease. Co-workers and patients may increasingly desire to not work with the individual.

Knowing the signs of alcohol abuse is the first step an organization and its managers can take in helping the troubled employee. A number of companies have reported success with helping employees in well-run alcohol abuse programs. Among them is the Wausau Insurance Company whose program began in 1969 to provide assistance to employees who are experiencing problems with alcohol and drugs.[13] Increasingly, companies are instituting policies similar to the one in Figure 7-2. Here, the company is trying to provide preliminary assistance but retains the authority to terminate the employee if the individual repeatedly fails to comply.

Drug Abuse

As evidenced in the newspaper and on television, drug abuse is a growing problem in American society. The problems range from the overuse of legal drugs such as tranquilizers and barbiturates to the use of illegal drugs such as marijuana, cocaine, and heroin. Of the drugs most readily available, cocaine is recognized as the fastest-growing form of American drug abuse.

One of the many potential causes for drug abuse is the stress the individual perceives that is coming from the job. Employees may abuse drugs as a way of temporarily escaping problems they have at home or boredom they have on the job. Whatever the reasons, drug abuse can be dangerous to the employee and costly to the health care organization. Actual cases involving drug abuse include:[14]

- A construction worker dies after falling eight stories. The autopsy showed the individual had smoked marijuana on the job.
- A forklift operator smokes marijuana on the job and then proceeds to run a forklift loaded with cargo into a door.
- A wallstreet trader made an $18 million trade and cannot recall the incident because of a cocaine-clouded memory.

The first step in dealing with a potential drug abuse problem is to realize it may be job related. Management should look for ways to reduce

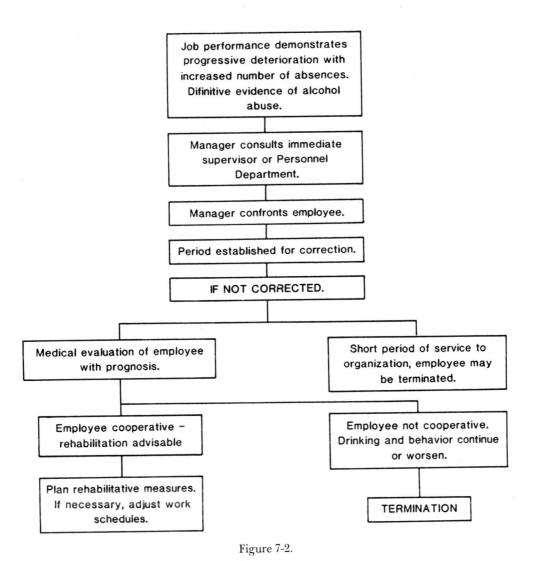

Figure 7-2.

stress and develop policies and procedures for effectively handling the problems once they arise. Health care organizations must be particularly careful, since the lives of patients may be endangered if wrong decisions are made as a direct result of employee-related drug abuse. To prevent problems, organizations should try to screen out prospective employees who are abusing drugs and develop plans for handling employees who develop a drug problem later on. Basic requirements for a drug prevention and abuse program should include:

1) Developing selection procedures to screen out those persons who

abuse drugs. Testing procedures may involve sample blood and urine tests.

2) Develop policies and procedures to cope with a drug abuse problem once it has been identified.

Some companies have aggressively begun to remove employees once it has been determined there is a drug or alcohol abuse problem. The following is representative of how some companies have reacted to evidence of employee drug abuse.[15]

- Blue Cross and Blue Shield of Boston terminated 21 workers after it had been determined they were using drugs at work.
- The Burns International Company terminated 21 unarmed guards at a California Nuclear Plant after they either refused to take or failed urine tests.
- The Shell Oil Company now conducts random drug searches on workers going on and off duty aboard drilling platforms.
- The National Transportation and Safety Board found that during an eleven-month period, seven train accidents involved either drug or alcohol use.

To combat the increasing problems with drug and alcohol abuse, many companies have developed comprehensive assistance programs. The Employee Assistance Program (EAP's) is an example of one such program. Here, the employer establishes a liaison relationship with a social service counseling agency. When the employee or employer recognizes the potential problem, the individual is referred to the counseling organization. Costs for the counseling services are paid by the employing organization in total or to a pre-established limit. Providing such a program helps an organization develop good employee relations and is good for the United States economy. Some estimates place the cost of drug abuse at $60 billion annually.

ORGANIZATIONAL POLICIES ON ALCOHOL AND DRUG ABUSE

All health care organizations should have policies on how to handle employee alcohol and drug abuse. The problems employees have should be dealt with individually and in a consistent manner. One such policy, developed by the Kemper Insurance Group, is an industry model for how to manage alcoholism, drug abuse, or emotional disturbances. The Kemper policy is as follows:

Kemper Insurance Group Personnel Assistance Policy Statement

POLICY. The underlying concept of Kemper's personnel policies is regard for the employee as an individual as well as a worker. Reflecting this concern, the company has devised a policy with six principles.[16]

1) We believe that alcoholism, drug addiction, and emotional disturbance are illnesses and should be treated as such.
2) We believe the majority of employees who develop alcoholism, other drug addiction or emotional illness can be helped to recover and the company should offer appropriate assistance.
3) We believe the decision to seek diagnosis and accept treatment for any suspected illness is the responsibility of the employee. However, continued refusal of an employee to seek treatment when it appears that substandard performance may be caused by an illness is not tolerated. We believe that alcoholism, other drug addiction or emotional illness should not be made an exception to this commonly accepted principle.
4) We believe that it is in the best interest of employees and the company that when alcoholism, other drug addictions, or emotional illness is present, it should be diagnosed and treated at the earliest possible date.
5) We believe that the company's concern for the individual alcohol drinking, drug taking, and behavioral habits begins only when they result in unsatisfactory job performance, poor attendance or behavior detrimental to the good reputation of the companies.
6) We believe that confidential handling of the diagnosis and treatment of alcoholism, other drug addictions or emotional illness is essential.

The objective of the Kemper policy is to retain employees who have developed any of these illnesses. The attempt is to arrest the condition before it renders them unemployable.

THE SUPERVISOR'S RESPONSIBILITY IN ALCOHOL AND DRUG ABUSE PROBLEMS

Health care managers are hired by organizations to monitor and direct employee performance. Supervisors should not become self-proclaimed experts in the diagnosis of either drug or alcohol problems. Above all, the director of physical therapy should not become a counselor in a situation where an employee has such an illness. Few physical therapists possess the background for handling these types of problems. The best solution is to approach the employee's problem just as you would with any other problem with employee performance.

Suspected instances of alcohol and drug abuse should be carefully documented. Once the problem more clearly manifests itself, all incidents of inappropriate behavior should be recorded so the employee can be confronted. When the employee is confronted, it must be in a manner which outlines the unacceptable behavior and specifies how it is to be improved. A time limit should be set which reinforces the importance of correcting the behavior.

Once discovered, the employee may begin an attempt to conceal the problem and further deny its existence. It is not uncommon for the employee to try and leave the appearance of doing a better job than ever before. If performance continues to deteriorate, the supervisor should once again confront the employee. This time the confrontation must be more direct and specifically point out the unsatisfactory performance. Asking for a resignation may be an effective way to stimulate the employee to recognize the problem. Employees rarely like losing a job over alcohol or drug abuse, since it is seldom easy to find another. Remember, above all, it is the supervisor's job to uncover the poor performance, not to become a diagnostician of possible alcohol or drug dependency.

PERSONAL AND ORGANIZATIONAL WAYS TO REDUCE STRESS

The health care manager is the individual who is in the best position to reduce the stress associated with working in an organization. It is important to point out, however, that some of the methods chosen to reduce stress may work for one person but not for another. The following are a number of the most common methods to reduce stress for the individual and for the organization.

1) THE MANAGER MUST GIVE CAREFUL THOUGHT TO PLANNING. Proper planning helps avoid situations that produce high levels of stress. Health care management can be much easier when the physical therapist plans the department so that it operates in an organized fashion. The supervisor can begin by outlining what it is that he or she would like to accomplish on a particular day. Many

top executives begin each day by listing the activities which should be performed. Throughout the day, activities which are completed are crossed off the list. This helps avoid the haphazard movement from project to project without following anything through to the end. Figure 7-3 examines the performance stress relationship. The vertical axis demonstrates a level of performance which varies from low to high. The horizontal axis demonstrates the amount of stress which can also vary from low to high. At low stress levels the job may be of little challenge and subsequently be stressful. As indicated by the curve, increasing levels of stress can improve performance up to a point, after which it will begin to deteriorate. At high levels of stress, employees are unable to perform at their best.

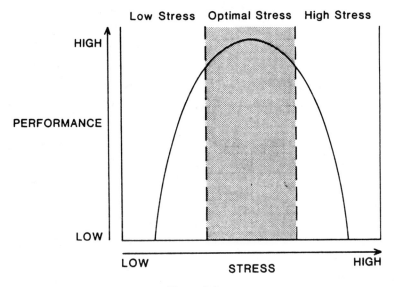

Figure 7-3.

2) MANAGE A SITUATION WITH THE IDEA OF CONTROLLING THE LEVEL OF STRESS. Too often, the inexperienced health care manager will try and do it all. In most cases, the attempts to do it all are not an exercise power and control but an internalized belief that no one else can do the job as well as the supervisor. Another common reason is that the manager feels inexperienced with delegating. One of the best ways for the manager to reduce personal and organizational stress is to delegate. The extent to which a manager

delegates authority to perform a task is influenced by a variety of factors. Some of the most common factors include the culture of the organization, the situation, the relationships, personalities, and the capabilities of the people in the situation.[17]

When properly used, the supervisor's option to delegate work to subordinates provides a number of advantages. One of the most important advantages is the time it makes available for the pursuit of other activities. With free time available as a result of the delegation, the manager can then accept assignments of greater importance to higher level managers. It is important to remember, however, the manager should not just delegate routine assignments but also those that require creative thinking. This helps to relieve the manager of having to think about complex responsibilities while also providing employees with an opportunity to exercise creative thinking.

Another advantage of delegation is that it frequently leads to better decisions. Those employees who are close to the problem are more likely to have a better understanding of the situation. For example, rather than implementing a complex policy and procedure for hydrotherapy, as a result of a patient fall, the manager should consult with employees who were present at the time when the patient fell. The supervisor should ask for their recommendations on how to avoid future problems. These same employees may be provided with guidelines on policy and procedure development and asked to develop some for actual implementation.

Delegation is also a time-saver. When employees are given the authority and responsibility for a task, they make decisions regarding how it should be completed. This saves time, since the subordinate does not have to check with the supervisor before making each decision. A health care manager must be willing to accept the fact that there are a number of ways to perform a given task. A subordinate may choose one way which is opposite of the way the supervisor would have proceeded. It should be assumed that subordinates will make errors in judgment. The supervisor should, however, provide an opportunity for them to learn from their mistakes. Those managers who encourage subordinates to use their abilities will find subordinates who are more committed to task accomplishment and more likely to accept responsibility for an outcome.

3) RELAX IN PRESSURE SITUATIONS. Relaxing in pressure situations is obviously much easier said than done. Much of the anxiety the individual perceives is as a result of a fear of the unknown or the fear of failure. Knowing your individual capabilities is the first step to relaxing in pressure situations. If you have confidence in your professional training and your ability to supervise health care professionals, you should have little, if any, problem in management. Always be honest and straightforward with subordinates about your background as a supervisor. Quite often, subordinates will be of assistance to those individuals new to health care management.

4) QUANTITATIVE AND QUALITATIVE JOB OVERLOAD. When quantitative overload occurs, the supervisor must evaluate how effectively human and non-human resources are being utilized. If the volume of patients seen in the department is increasing, the supervisor must encourage the administration to recruit additional staff. If the department is properly staffed, the supervisor should evaluate the methods of organization. Lack of delegation may be the problem.

Qualitative overload can be reduced by slowing the pace of managerial decision making. If the manager feels as though decision making is rushed, it is better to postpone the decision until more information is available. Those therapists new to health care management should strive to make correct decisions over quick decisions. Making correct decisions may be more time consuming but can be beneficial in building managerial self-confidence.

UNDERUTILIZATION OF ABILITIES AND ROLE AMBIGUITY

Physical therapists who accept directors' positions in small hospitals often verbalize that their talents and abilities are not being utilized to the fullest. Rather than allowing the job to become monotonous, the supervisor should look for ways to provide personal job challenge as well as challenge for the employee. Job enrichment is one way to solve many of the problems health care managers face today concerning job dissatisfaction. Management must recognize that the nature of a job has a powerful effect on individual motivation. Job enrichment is an approach to increasing motivation and productivity by making basic changes to the job.

A job that is considered enriched is one which is characterized by increased responsibility, personal achievement, recognition, and individual growth. Fredrick Herzberg originally set forth the concepts of job enrichment.[18] They are:

- Frequent feedback of performance results.
- Opportunity to perceive psychological growth.
- Opportunity to schedule one's own work.
- Employee responsibility for some job costs.
- A flexible managerial hierarchy.
- Employee accountability for results.

More recently, Hackman and Oldham identified experienced meaningfulness, experienced responsibility, and knowledge of results as essentials for enriched jobs.[19] For subordinates, an enriched job provides feedback and allows participation in decision making, problem solving, and goal setting. At the level of supervisor, the individual must develop and implement plans which allow the department and organization to function more smoothly. Following through on plans, such as designing and building a new department, provides the supervisor with increased responsibility, achievement, goal accomplishment, and recognition from top management for a job well done. Figure 7-4 illustrates the basic concepts of the Hackman/Oldham theory of job enrichment.

According to their research, supervisors can take the initiative to enrich their own jobs and the jobs of subordinates. The key variables for job enrichment are defined as follows:

- EXPERIENCED MEANINGFULNESS. This is the degree to which work is recognized as important, worthwhile, and valuable.
- EXPERIENCED RESPONSIBILITY. The extent to which the individual feels personally responsible for the job being performed.
- KNOWLEDGE OF RESULTS. The degree to which an employee receives feedback about job performance.

    The psychological states are affected by the characteristics of the tasks subordinates are performing. They are:

- SKILL VARIETY. The degree to which a job requires the use of several skills or talents in the performance of an activity.
- TASK IDENTITY. The degree to which the employee completes a whole piece of work. This is the opportunity to see the job to a final outcome.

JOB CHARACTERISTICS - MODEL OF MOTIVATION

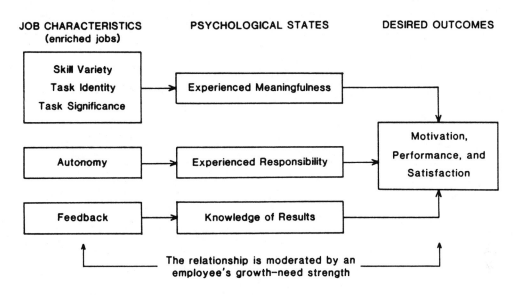

Figure 7-4.

- TASK SIGNIFICANCE. The degree to which the job has an impact on others and the organization.

The individual's ability to experience responsibility is related to autonomy.

- AUTONOMY. The degree to which the job provides freedom in scheduling work and in carrying out problems.

The level of feedback affects the individual's knowledge of results.

- FEEDBACK. The degree to which task completion provides the individual with information about the effectiveness of performance.

As noted in Figure 7-4, growth-need strength is the individual's need for personal accomplishment as well as the creativity of the job. An employee who has little need for growth may be dissatisfied with an enriched job. Those employees who have a need to grow will be motivated by jobs which have the five important characteristics. To properly use the model calls for the supervisor to diagnose the employee's growth-need strength. Through a better understanding of what affects employee motivation, the supervisor can better tailor the job to the individual.

One of the primary advantages of job enrichment is that it helps involve employees in decision making and satisfies their needs for responsibility, achievement, and recognition. Jobs which have little or no enrichment will be more stressful, since they tend to communicate that employees are irresponsible, unmotivated, and incapable of learning or growing on the job. The following principles will provide further assistance in making jobs more challenging and less stressful.

1) REMOVE SOME OF THE CONTROLS. Allow employees some flexibility in deciding how a job should be done rather than having exact methods dictated to them.

2) MAKE EMPLOYEES PERSONALLY ACCOUNTABLE. Job enrichment specifies that employees should be responsible for the results they obtain. The job should provide some level of feedback concerning the performance obtained.

3) PROVIDE NATURAL WORK UNITS. The most rewarding settings in which to provide patient care are those which allow the professional to follow the rehabilitation of the patient from beginning to end. Encourage the staff to periodically re-evaluate the progress of patients weeks or even months after final discharge.

4) DELEGATE AUTHORITY AS INDICATED. As the individual grows in their ability to perform a job, increase their authority to act as needed. Allow employees to decide what information is needed to do a job, and provide the opportunity for them to obtain the information without having to go through formal channels.

5) PROVIDE REGULAR PERFORMANCE EVALUATIONS. The employee should be informed, on a regular basis, how their work is proceeding. If performance is in need of adjustment, the supervisor should provide only an outline as to how it should be corrected. The employee should be allowed to fill in the details.

Instances of role ambiguity can be a particular problem to a health care manager. When the manager receives confusing or conflicting signals from top management, the result will be increased levels of personal stress. When your job and the responsibilities you assume are in a continual state of flux, meet with your supervisor and discuss the situation. If your job is confusing, it could be the result of your supervisor's failure to outline what is expected.

MANAGERIAL AND ORGANIZATIONAL STRATEGIES FOR COPING WITH STRESS

There are a number of managerial approaches to helping reduce the level of stress in organizations.[20] The health care manager must begin by analyzing the sources of stress and understanding the factors that contribute to job tension. Once the sources have been determined, managers can work in developing approaches to help the individual control the source of stress in the job. In some organizations where stress is a particular problem, top management has started including stress management training for supervisors and their employees.

Stress can be partially alleviated through the manager's willingness to listen. When listening to what an employee has to say the manager should avoid practicing psychotherapy or psychiatry. It is not the manager's role to offer advice on personal problems but instead to aid in the development of work-oriented problem solving. Whenever an employee presents a psychological problem, encourage the individual to seek professional help. Remember, as a health care manager, only offer assistance in areas where you consider yourself competent.

Finally, managers should allow employees greater participation in decision making. A subordinate who has an opportunity to participate in decision making is likely to have a more positive view of the organization. When employee opinions, knowledge, and desires are excluded from the organizational decision-making process, the resulting lack of participation can lead to increased strain and reduced productivity.[21] Managers who are aware of the causes and consequences of stress can reduce job tension and create a more satisfying work environment.

REFERENCES

1. S. A. Yolles, "Mental Health at Work." In A. McLean (ed.), To Work is Human: Mental Health and the Business Community (New York: Macmillan, 1967.)
2. The discussion of these factors in work stress is based in part on J. E. McGrath, "Stress and Behavior in Organizations," in Handbook in Industrial and Organizational Psychology, ed. M. D. Dunnette (Chicago, IL: Rand McNally, 1976), pp. 1351–1395.
3. See, for example, J. R. P. French and R. D. Caplan, "Organizational Stress and Individual Strain," in The Failure of Success, ed. A. J. Marrow (New York: AMA–COM, 1972); S. Parasuraman and A. J. Alutto, "An Examina-

tion of the Organizational Antecedents of Stressors at Work," Academy of Management Journal, 24, (1981); pp. 48–67; and A. Zaleznick, M.F.R. Kets de Vries, and J. Howard, "Stress Reactions in Organizations; Syndromes, Causes, and Consequences," Behavioral Science, 22 (1977), pp. 151–162.

4. V. A. Price, Type A Behavior Pattern (New York: Academic Press, 1982), p. 3

5. M. Friedman and R. H. Rosenman, Type A Behavior and Your Heart (New York: Alfred A. Knopf, 1974).

6. The comparisons between type A and type B individuals are based on A. A. McLean, Work Stress (Reading, MA: Addison-Wesley, 1979), pp. 68–71.

7. T. Cox, Stress (Baltimore: University Park Press, 1978), p. 92.

8. J. D. Kearns, Stress in Industry (London: Priory Press, 1973).

9. J. F. McKenna, P. L. Oritt, and H. K. Wolff, "Occupational Stress as a Predictor in the Turnover Decision," Journal of Human Stress, December 1981, pp. 12–17.

10. O. A. Parsons, "Alcoholics' Neuropsychological Impairment: Current Findings and Conclusions," Annals of Behavior Medicine, (March 1986), pp. 13–19.

11. J. C. Finney, D. F. Smith, D. E. Skeeters, and C. Auvenshine, "MMPI and Alcoholic Scales," Quarterly Journal of Studies on Alcohol (November 1971), pp. 1055–1060.

12. M. B. Sobell and L. C. Sobell, "Functional Analysis of Alcohol Problems," in Medical Psychology: Contributions to Behavioral Medicine, ed. C. K. Prokop and L. A. Bradley (New York: Academic Press, 1981), pp. 81–90.

13. H. B. Preston and M. E. Bierman, "An Insurance Company's EAP Produces Results," November–December 1985, EAP Digest, pp. 21–28.

14. "Taking Drugs on the Job," Newsweek (August 22, 1982, p. 52.)

15. C. W. English, "Getting Tough on Worker Abuse of Drugs, Alcohol," U.S. News & World Report (December 5, 1983), p. 85.

16. Frederick Willman and Mark Ellen Kane, The Kemper Approach to Alcoholism, Drug Addiction, and Other Living Problems (Kemper Group, Long Grove, IL, 1986), pp. 12–13.

17. See Gerald G. Fisch, "Toward Effective Delegation," CPA Journal, 46, no. 7 (July 1976): pp. 66–67.

18. Fredrick Herzberg, "Orthodox Job Enrichment: A Common Sense Approach to People at Work," Defense Management Journal, April 1977, pp. 21–27.

19. J. R. Hackman and G. Oldham, Work Redesign (Reading, MA: Addison-Wesley, 1980).

20. For additional approaches to deal with job stress, see: Gary L. Cooper and Roy Payne, Stress at Work (New York: John Wiley & Sons, 1978); Rosalind Forbes, Corporate Stress: How to Manage on the Job and Make it Work for You (New York: Doubleday and Co., 1979), Alan A. McLean, Work Stress, (Reading, MA: Addison-Wesley, 1979) and Arthur P. Brief, Randall S. Schuler and Mary Van Sell, Managing Job Stress (Boston: Little, Brown and Co., 1981).

21. L. Coch & J. R. P. French, "Overcoming Resistance to Change," Human Relations, 1948, 1, pp. 512–533.

Chapter Eight

MANAGING CONFLICT AND FRUSTRATION IN HEALTH CARE ORGANIZATIONS

DEFINING AND RECOGNIZING CONFLICT
  Intrapersonal Conflict
  Interpersonal Conflict
  Intragroup Conflict
  Intergroup Conflict
  Intraorganizational Conflict
  Interorganizational Conflict
METHODS FOR REDUCING INTERGROUP CONFLICT
  Avoidance
  Defusion
  Confrontation
COPING WITH FRUSTRATION
CONSTRUCTIVE AND DISRUPTIVE RESULTS OF FRUSTRATION
UTILIZING DEFENSE MECHANISMS
CONFLICT, FRUSTRATION, AND HUMAN RELATIONS

Health care managers are increasingly concerned about the level of conflict present in their organizations. Conflict is an important issue to health care organizations and should be recognized as arising from any number of diverse causes. Anytime health care professionals and groups interact with one another there are bound to be differences of opinion. Differences of opinion will naturally occur at all levels in the organizational hierarchy.

With the levels of conflict increasing there is a greater desire by managers to know more about it and how it should be properly managed. A recent survey indicates that middle and top managers report spending approximately 20 percent of their time dealing directly with some form of conflict.[1] With the increasing amounts of time being devoted to conflict resolution, conflict skills are becoming more important to the job of the health care manager.

Management has historically viewed conflict in two different ways. Traditionally, conflict was viewed as destructive and was something which was to be avoided at all costs. Conflict is still considered as undesirable for the following reasons:[2]

1) Conflict produces high levels of stress for those directly and indirectly involved. It can interrupt decision processes and result in discontent and frustration.

2) Conflict disrupts social groups. People who are members of groups are told it is important to get along with others and to avoid conflict.

3) Managerial effectiveness is often evaluated by the degree of harmony present within the department and the organization. Rewards are often based on how well everyone gets along.

The traditional view of conflict sees any type of conflict as potentially destructive and deserving of elimination. Its primary causes are from personality conflicts or from the failure of managerial leadership. According to the traditional view, conflict should be resolved by physically separating the parties or by direct management intervention. The traditional approach assumes conflict will not occur if sound management principles are applied to designing and directing the organization. The idea is that if conflict does occur, management can take the appropriate steps and resolve the matter quickly.

A second view of conflict, the contemporary view, recognizes conflict as a consequence of everyday organizational life. Conflict may not only be inevitable, it may also be desirable and help to stimulate organizational change.[3] One study indicated that conflict among established groups tended to improve performance in comparison to when there was no conflict at all.[4]

The health care manager must realize that conflict can have a positive or negative effect on performance, depending on how it is managed.[5] The constructive aspects of conflict will result in better organizational performance. Conflict is recognized as dysfunctional when it hinders the attainment of organizational objectives and goals. As shown in Figure 8-1, conflict can be considered functional or potentially as a threat to organizational survival.

CONSTRUCTIVE CONFLICT

1) Problems between profesionals are identified.

2) The members of the department are stimulated.

3) Creativity may be encouraged in the professional.

4) Members may become more committed to goals.

DESTRUCTIVE CONFLICT

1) Cooperation is reduced.

2) Group goals are replaced by individual goals.

3) Stress levels increase in the department or organization.

4) Competition lessens cooperation.

Figure 8-1.

DEFINING AND RECOGNIZING CONFLICT

There are many ways by which to recognize and define conflict. A person may experience conflict in the form of an argument, contradiction, or incompatibility. As such, conflict may be defined as any situation in which there are incompatible goals or emotions within or between groups. Conflict has also been defined as a process which begins when one party perceives that the other has frustrated, or is about to frustrate, some concern.[6] In other words, conflict occurs whenever goal-directed behavior of one person or group is blocked by another person or group. Each of these definitions recognize three basic types of conflict.

1) GOAL CONFLICT. A form of conflict which occurs when desired outcomes are incompatible.
2) COGNITIVE CONFLICT. The psychological state of the individual where thought patterns or ideas are seemingly inconsistent.
3) AFFECTIVE CONFLICT. A form of conflict where emotions or feelings are incompatible with one another. This is a situation where people literally become angry at one another.

Within and outside of the organization different levels of conflict exist. The six levels of conflict are: intrapersonal (within the individual), interpersonal (between individuals), intragroup (within a group), intergroup (between groups), intraorganizational (within an organization), and interorganizational (between organizations). Figure 8-2 portrays the differences.

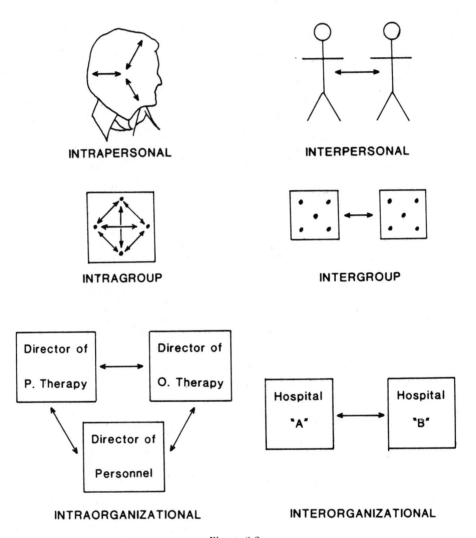

INTRAPERSONAL   INTERPERSONAL

INTRAGROUP   INTERGROUP

INTRAORGANIZATIONAL   INTERORGANIZATIONAL

Figure 8-2.

Intrapersonal Conflict

Intrapersonal conflict occurs within the individual most often involving a goal or cognitive conflict. In the goal conflict situation a certain behavior will result in outcomes that are: (a) mutually exclusive or (b) have incompatible elements (both positive and negative outcomes). In other words, there may be positive, negative, or combination of outcomes. Three types of interpersonal goal conflict can be identified.

1) Approach-Approach Conflict

In this form of conflict situation the person has a choice between two or more positive alternatives. The person may, for example, have a choice between two equally promising jobs. The individual must choose between the two or more courses of action and reject all others. The approach-approach situation seldom results in high levels of tension or frustration, because all of the alternatives are considered rewarding. The choice between alternatives occasionally takes longer if the alternatives are seen as having equal value.

2) Approach-Avoidance Conflict

The individual may be placed in a situation which presents both positive and negative consequences. A therapist may, for example, be offered an excellent job in an area of the country the individual considers undesirable. The goal of obtaining a challenging job may be positive, but the behavior required to achieve the goal has negative consequences.

3) Avoidance-Avoidance Conflict

Here, the individual must choose between two or more negative alternatives. An employee may be forced to choose between the loss of a job or accepting a reduction in pay. Ideally, the person would like to physically avoid either of the alternatives.

Intrapersonal cognitive conflict results from inconsistencies in an individual's thought processes. The thought process can include beliefs about their own behavior, environment, or about themselves. Inconsistent beliefs or thoughts are psychologically uncomfortable for most people. According to the Theory of Cognitive Dissonance, the inconsistencies and discomfort produced usually helps to motivate the individual to reduce the level of inconsistency.[7] Those who experience discomfort are motivated to reduce the dissonance (inconsistency) and achieve a state of consonance (equilibrium). To achieve a state of equilibrium the person can either change their beliefs or obtain more information about the issue causing dissonance.

Interpersonal Conflict

Interpersonal conflict concerns the method and quality of interactions between two individuals. People respond to interpersonal conflict based on either a desire to satisfy their own concerns, the concerns of others, or some combination of the two extremes. The desire to satisfy personal goals depends on the extent to which the person is assertive. A person who desires to satisfy the concerns of others has a more cooperative orientation. Five interpersonal conflict handling styles have been identified. They are:[8]

Avoidance Style

The person using this style is unassertive and uncooperative. The individual tries to stay out of conflicts by ignoring disagreements or by remaining neutral. The person may use this approach in the hopes the conflict will work itself out.

Forcing Style

The person who demonstrates the forcing style is assertive and reflects a win-lose approach to interpersonal conflict. These people are often concerned with their own goals and not those of others. The forcing style may involve elements of power and dominance and may result in unfavorable evaluations by others.

Accommodating Style

The accommodating style of managing interpersonal conflict is one in which the individual lacks assertiveness concerning their own choice of an outcome. Accommodation may be an attempt to encourage cooperation by the other person or a simple submission. The person who is accommodating is often evaluated favorably but may be perceived as weak.

Collaborative Style

The collaborative style reflects a win-win approach to interpersonal conflict. The individual will evidence behavior that is both assertive and cooperative. Those who demonstrate the collaborative style desire to maximize joint outcomes. They present the following characteristics:[9]

- They do not see conflict as negative but rather as natural. If managed properly, they see conflict as leading to more creative solutions.

- They trust and are open with others.
- They recognize that conflict which is resolved to the satisfaction of all parties is more likely to gain individual commitment.
- Each member is considered as having an equal stake in helping to solve the conflict.
- No one is sacrificed simply for the good of the group.

Compromise Style

The compromise style represents a behavior which falls between being cooperative and that of being assertive. People who compromise do not tend to maximize joint satisfaction. Each person receives only partial satisfaction based on a give-and-take process. The use of the compromise style typically involves negotiation and a series of concessions.

The Result of Interpersonal Conflict Handling Styles

Research into interpersonal conflict handling styles indicates that most people use collaboration as a means of resolving their conflicts.[10] Collaboration is more representative of:

1) Successful Managers
2) Higher Performing Organizations

People who utilize the collaborative style of conflict resolution are perceived as dynamic individuals who use conflict constructively. Collaborative people have more positive feelings about themselves and traditionally receive positive feedback from others. In contrast to the collaborating style, the forcing and avoiding techniques tend to be associated with unfavorable self-evaluations, negative feelings from others, and a general lack of the constructive use of conflict. Accommodating and compromising appear to produce only mixed results. Based on the available findings, the collaborative style appears to be the best for managing interpersonal conflict.

Intragroup Conflict

Intragroup conflict concerns conflict within a group as well as between individuals. The conflict situation will affect how the group operates, its outputs, and its social processes. Groups experiencing conflict may resolve it or not, depending on the depth of the disagreement among members. A study involving groups in business and government identified some of the conditions that lead to successful and unsuccessful conflict resolution.[11] The study indicated that intragroup conflicts seems to fall into two categories: substantive conflict and affective conflict.

Substantive conflict is a conflict based on the task which the group performs or to "content" issues. There will be intellectual disagreements between and among members. Affective conflict is associated with emotional responses from interpersonal relations. The study demonstrated that a group experiencing substantive conflict achieves consensus by emphasizing positive factors that help to promote consensus. A group experiencing affective conflict achieves consensus by reducing the negative forces that promote disagreement.

Intergroup Conflict

Intergroup conflict occurs between two or more groups. Although not as common in the health care environment, groups may occasionally compete with one another over scarce resources or because of differences in opinion. Intergroup conflict can stimulate competition which leads to improved performance. Intergroup competition should not, however, be allowed to continue to the point where the losing group becomes demoralized and adopts a defeatist attitude.

Intraorganizational Conflict

Intraorganizational conflict can occur within an organization in any one of four ways. Intraorganizational conflict is seen as: (1) vertical conflict, (2) horizontal conflict, (3) line-staff conflict, or (4) role conflict. Each of the four types of intraorganizational conflicts have distinct characteristics.

Vertical conflict refers to a situation involving conflict between different levels within the organization's hierarchy. Vertical conflicts often arise when supervisors attempt to control subordinates and subordinates resist their control efforts.[12] Inadequate or poor communication, conflicts of interest, and a lack of consensus concerning the meaning of information or values can also cause vertical conflict.[13]

Horizontal conflict occurs between departments or employees on the same organizational level. The primary reason for horizontal conflict is from suboptimalization. A department may seek its own goals over the goals of another department. As such, the goals may be incompatible between departments. The perception created is one which leads to conflict between departments.

Line-staff conflict is not as frequently seen in the health care organization as it is in business and industry. Hospitals have staff departments, such as personnel, to assist the line departments such as physical therapy, occupational therapy, and the department of x-ray. A line manager such as the director of physical therapy is responsible for managing the daily activities of a department. The staff manager serves in an advisory capacity to assist the line manager.

Staff managers often present a different set of personality characteristics than line managers. Those individuals occupying staff positions often have higher levels of education, different backgrounds, and are younger than line employees.[14] The differences in values and characteristics set up the potential for conflict to develop. It is not uncommon for line managers to express feeling as though staff members are infringing on their authority.

Role conflict is a stress resulting from incompatible messages a person receives concerning the cluster of activities others expect them to perform. Those people in role sender positions have expectations and perceptions of the focal person's activities. These expectations influence the messages which are transmitted. A focal person's role set includes the manager, subordinates, and other employees with whom the person works. Conflict can result when the focal person receives incompatible messages and pressures from the role set. Daniel Katz and Robert L. Kahn identified six types of role conflict.[15] They are:

1) INTRASENDER CONFLICT. Here a single supervisor provides a subordinate with a set of incompatible orders or expectations.

2) INTERSENDER CONFLICT. Occurs when the expectations from one person or group differ with the expectations of another person or group. Two individuals or groups may be sending the focal person different messages.

3) INTER-ROLE CONFLICT. A type of conflict that often creates tension in both the job and home, especially in two-career families.[16] The person is expected to play different roles which give rise to conflicting demands. Typically, the pressures associated with membership in one group conflicts with the pressures from membership in another group.

4) PERSON-ROLE CONFLICT. This form of conflict occurs when job

requirements run opposite to individual values or needs. A physical therapist may, for example, feel uncomfortable working in a physician's office if the person is strongly against referral for profit. The salary offered may, however, make it difficult to refuse the opportunity.

5) ROLE OVERLOAD CONFLICT. Here the person is confronted with expectations from a number of sources which cannot be completed in a given period of time and still maintain quality. The therapist who has thirty patients to see in eight hours may be concerned over the quality of health care services offered.

6) ROLE AMBIGUITY. In this situation the individual is uncertain about what is to be done since insufficient information has been provided about job responsibilities.

Unmanaged role conflict undermines effectiveness in the organization. The important task for management is to maintain role conflict at an optimal level and avoid situations which produce dysfunctional conflict. The manager must aim at promoting a positive organizational atmosphere while minimizing the negative or dysfunctional effects that unmanaged role conflict can produce.

Interorganizational Conflict

Interorganizational conflict is that which occurs between organizations. Many consider the conflict which occurs between organizations as a form of healthy competition. The external environment is becoming increasingly more competitive, especially at the hospital level. The National Association for Ambulatory Care estimates that 2,600 centers were in operation by July of 1985.[17] They estimate that a new center is being added at the rate of one per day. Patients are reshaping the way medicine is practiced and how organizations operate. Interorganizational conflict will continue and probably increase as long as each organization must continue to scramble for every health care dollar.

METHODS FOR REDUCING INTERGROUP CONFLICT

Conflict is undoubtedly a fact of life in today's complex health care organization. The physical therapy supervisor must be prepared to resolve conflict before dysfunctional consequences affect the department and the organization's performance. Conflict management is an important but often difficult skill for the manager to develop. The methods for effectively resolving intergroup conflict can be broken down into three classifications. They are avoidance, defusion, and confrontation.[18] Each of these and their various subclassifications is discussed as follows:

Avoidance

The avoidance of conflict is evidenced when a manager does not want to confront a problem. The lack of desire to confront the problem may be as a result of a number of reasons. The manager may believe the issue is trivial and feel other issues are more deserving of attention. Other reasons may be that the manager will try and let subordinates resolve it themselves before attempting to seek a solution. The avoidance style of conflict resolution can be broken down into three areas: non-attention, physical separation, and limited interaction.

Non-attention is a situation where the manager totally ignores the problem or potential source of conflict. Here, the manager hopes that time will provide an effective solution for the problem. Depending on the severity of the situation, non-attention may allow the conflict to resolve itself effectively. In other cases, the problem may disappear for a short period of time and then return. Conflict situations which repeatedly arise can seldom be managed by non-attention.

Physical separation is the process of actually separating the groups so they have literally no contact with one another. The theory behind physical separation is that people or groups who are not together cannot quarrel. This is, at best, only a temporary solution, since most health care organizations do not have the facility design to keep people apart. The physical separation of employees also tends to limit the organization's overall effectiveness because of the resources which must be committed to keep the groups apart.

Limited interaction is not as drastic as physical separation. Here, the manager tries to separate the groups so that they have limited contact with one another. In limited interactions the parties do see one another but only under formal situations, such as a meeting, where a strict agenda is to be followed. Limited interaction provides the same dysfunctional consequences as physical separation.

Defusion

The defusion strategy allows a period for "cool down" so the conflict situation becomes less emotional. The intent of the defusion strategy is to allow the parties to regain their perspective of the issue. The involved groups may come to an agreement on the small points concerning an issue and leave the major points for discussion at a later date. The theory when using this strategy is that the major points will diminish with time. The two methods of defusion are smoothing and compromise.

Smoothing is a diplomatic way of suppressing the conflict. The manager minimizes the extent and importance of the disagreement and tries to stress the similarities and common interests between the conflicting parties. The idea is to eventually lead the groups to the realization that they are not as far apart as they initially believed.

Compromise is a situation in which the manager attempts to resolve the conflict by convincing both parties that the object of desire or goal can be achieved in a way that both parties can live with. The managerial use of compromise can be an effective means of conflict resolution when the two groups are fairly equal in strength.

Confrontation

The confrontation method of resolving conflict provides an opportunity for the sources of conflict to be discussed, with an emphasis on satisfying the common interests of the parties. The most popular method of confrontation resolution is problem solving.

Problem solving provides an opportunity for both parties to work together to find a solution which is mutually acceptable. Problem solving includes the following steps:

1) DEFINE THE PROBLEM. Both parties must come to an agreement as to what the problem is.
2) A SEARCH FOR SOLUTIONS. Here the groups list and discuss the potential solutions. The role of the manager is to encourage the free flow of ideas. Each potential solution should be expressed without intimidation or criticism from other group members.
3) NARROW THE CHOICES. The groups may narrow the possible solutions to one or two and then reach a final consensus through voting. Secret ballot is recommended, since it eliminates the opportunity for individual member intimidation.

4) IMPLEMENT THE DECISION. Strive to gain the commitment of all group members by reminding them that the decision was reached through consensus.

5) EVALUATE THE RESULTS. Feedback helps reinforce the positive and negative aspects of a group decision.

Minimizing intergroup conflict is directly related to improving interpersonal relations within groups. The efforts to reduce conflict should not be so intense that they reduce the quality or quantity of health care services provided. Conflict can frequently lead to increased productivity as long as it is managed so that it does not create hostility and reduced organizational communication.

COPING WITH FRUSTRATION

Whenever a health care professional cannot achieve an objective, goal, promotion, pay raise, or other element of personal or professional importance, there is likely to be the development of frustration. An individual becomes frustrated when the desire to satisfy a need is blocked before the need can be satisfied. The individual may experience frustration due to an internal barrier, such as the tendency to procrastinate, or to an external barrier, such as the presence of substandard rehabilitation equipment. The key concept is that frustration is an individual perception. It is not considered a characteristic of the external environment.

In health care management, some level of frustration can be almost a daily event. Many health care professionals react to frustration by working harder or by encouraging others to work harder when objectives or goals have not been achieved. Whenever a person becomes frustrated, personal tension develops. The person develops tension when something or someone has thrown up a barrier which will not allow needs to be satisfied. Frustration on the job is most often the result of conflicts between what an individual wants and the restraints imposed by the health care organization. Depending upon the individual level of frustration, the person may demonstrate disruptive or aggressive behavior in reaction to real or imagined barriers blocking need satisfaction.

CONSTRUCTIVE AND DISRUPTIVE RESULTS OF FRUSTRATION

When a professional becomes frustrated, it is generally expected that the person will react in a negative way. Frustration can be a positive personal encounter if it is recognized as part of the job of the health care manager. Often, increased effort, choice of another goal, or rethinking the problem is all that is needed in order to relieve the sense of frustration. Encountering varying levels of personal frustration and managing them effectively is a required skill for top managers.

When frustration is not recognized by the health care manager as simply a barrier limiting the attainment of goals, it has the potential for becoming a destructive force. The individual may concentrate so intently on the unsuccessful attempt to reach the goal that other methods or goals are not considered. As such, the supervisor may lose the ability to deal constructively with the situation.

Some health care professions can tolerate higher levels of frustration than others. There are a number of factors which influence the individual's ability to deal with frustration. Among the most influential is the person's previous experience with the situation and how important the potential outcome was to the individual. Some people can tolerate a high degree of frustration for prolonged periods and still make realistic and rational choices. Others, depending on their background and experience, may panic and lose control. Recognizing how frustration is evidenced in the health care environment is important to the manager. Supervisory positions often contain more pressure, and subsequently more frustration, than their non-managerial counterparts. The two most common reactions to frustration are aggression and withdrawal.

Aggression involves a direct attack upon the person or barrier which is preventing attainment of the objective or goal. An individual who demonstrates aggression may do so physically, verbally, symbolically, or in a combination of ways. The supervisor who yells at an employee is demonstrating a verbal form of aggression. Aggression may also be displaced away from the object or person who created the sense of frustration. An individual may, for example, react with anger by kicking a trash can or by throwing a book. Aggression can be acted out in many forms, including theft, disobedience, sabotage, and absenteeism.

Aggression may also be withheld for prolonged periods until the person can find an appropriate means for expressing it. If for example, an employee were angry about the results of a performance evaluation it is unlikely the subordinate would yell at the supervisor. Demonstrating such behavior may get the person fired. The person may instead display antagonistic behavior or actively interfere with the work of others.

Physical or mental withdrawal is an attempt to reduce tension associated with a frustrating event by simply getting away from the area of concern. The person may withdraw temporarily or may do so permanently. Temporary withdrawal is demonstrated by a supervisor who is so frustrated with a situation or event that he or she simply walks away from the area of concern. Mentally, the person may "just want to forget about this for now." Withdrawal can also include the attitude of "I just don't care anymore." Those health care employees who repeatedly exhibit daydreaming characteristics may be psychologically withdrawing from a frustrating event or situation in their job.

UTILIZING DEFENSE MECHANISMS

Those individuals who continually physically or mentally withdraw from frustration may be demonstrating the use of defense mechanisms. Defense mechanisms make it possible for the person to temporarily reduce a level of tension. The use of a defense mechanism involves, to at least a certain degree, a distortion of the relationship the person has with external reality. Defense mechanisms allow the person to temporarily reduce tension but do not satisfy true underlying needs. Each of us, at one time or another, has witnessed defense mechanisms. As physical therapists, we often see patients demonstrate defense mechanisms when trying to justify continually missed appointments. The patient may use defense mechanisms to explain away the real reason for missed appointments. Knowing how to recognize defense mechanisms is the first step to helping the person cope with their usage and the frustration which created them. The most common types are: rationalization, repression, reaction formation, projection, identification, and regression.

Rationalization is the individual's attempt to explain away behaviors or outcomes that are undesirable or inconsistent. The explanations are an attempt to make the behavior or outcome acceptable or sometimes even bearable. The hospital employee who takes home surgical gowns for personal use may explain the theft by saying "everyone else in the department takes them home." Rationalization occurs when the person develops a "good reason" for a behavior or outcome rather than facing the unpleasant reality of the situation.

The two most common forms of rationalization are known as "sour grapes" and "sweet lemons." The individual who demonstrates sour grapes has convinced his or herself that the inability to obtain a valued object was not worth having anyhow. When the employee who was denied an important promotion states "the position wasn't that good for me anyhow, I'm above that sort of work," the person is displaying sour grapes.

Sweet lemons is a situation where the person convinces his or herself that an undesirable event is desirable. The physical therapist who repeatedly feels overworked may let the quality of patient care slip to the point where patients complain. The individual may be then heard to say, "Now maybe the hospital will listen to our requests to get more staff."

Reaction formation is demonstrated when the individual reacts by exhibiting the opposite attitudes and behavior to a desired area of concern. The employee who is angry at the supervisor may proceed to be so nice that it is almost intolerable. Here, the individual produces behavior that is opposite of the suppressed desire. The manager's attempt to diagnose reaction formation must proceed with caution. Knowledge of reaction formation is still quite limited; therefore, the health care manager must know a great deal about the employee before accurately determining whether the person is evidencing a reaction formation defense mechanism.

When the supervisor or one of the subordinates uses the repression form of defense mechanism the person unconsciously forgets painful or potentially frustrating information. Deliberate suppression of information is not the same as repression. Suppressing information is an attempt to hide something unpleasant. When the health care employee represses information it may be because of a fear of failure. The employee may, for example, forget to schedule a return visit for a patient who has repeatedly complained about past treatment results.

Projection is a process the individual uses to protect oneself from becoming aware of their own undesirable characteristics. Projection allows the person to attribute their own undesirable characteristics onto others. The supervisor who personally dislikes an employee may comment that the individual dislikes them. The supervisor may be overheard to say, "Why does so and so dislike me so much? What have I ever done?" Interestingly enough, individuals who are repeatedly turned down for promotions may believe others are out to get them rather than recognizing their own skills and abilities are the source of the problem.

Identification is a process whereby an individual assumes the values, attitudes, opinions, or behaviors of someone they admire. A subordinate may, for example, dress like the supervisor or begin to adopt mannerisms, speech, or social characteristics of the person they admire. The individual may not make an effort to acquire the same educational background or experience as the admired person but may, instead, be satisfied with being associated with someone they feel is rich or successful. A secretary may be so closely identified with the supervisor that he or she feels qualified to make decisions when the supervisor is absent.

Regression is behavior based on the individual's past and is recognized as a less than responsible behavior. Frustration can reach the point for some that they attempt to revert to an earlier and less mature behavior. In the midst of a frustrating job the person may decide to quit and go to an amusement park. Temper tantrums, pounding on the desk, or assuming child-like behavior are all forms of regression.

CONFLICT, FRUSTRATION, AND HUMAN RELATIONS

Each of us has demonstrated defense mechanisms during some point in our career. Defense mechanisms are helpful for coping with the variety of conflict situations and frustrating circumstances which arise in health care organizations. For the supervisor, it is important to understand that perceived stress, frustration and conflict are all reactions to situations occurring within the organization. The employee may be repeatedly arriving at work late because the individual finds the job dull and desires to avoid coming to work. The manager can only serve to compound the problem by scolding the worker for the chronic tardiness.

Defense mechanisms are normal reactions to situations that subordinates, supervisors and patients have when presented with uncomfortable or unfamiliar stimuli. Normally, defense mechanisms are not a problem unless they are continually relied upon. Becoming knowledgeable of defense mechanisms allows the supervisor to know more about him or herself and about others. Additionally, defense mechanisms provide clues about a worker's ability to handle delicate and complex situations. Understanding defense mechanisms is important for reducing on-the-job tension for both the manager and the subordinate.

REFERENCES

1. K. W. Thomas & W. H. Schmidt, "A Survey of Managerial Interests with Respect to Conflict," Academy of Management Journal, 1976, pp. 315–318.
2. S. P. Robbins, "Conflict Management and Conflict Resolutions Are Not Synonymous Terms," California Management Review, Winter 1978, pp. 67–75.
3. S. P. Robbins, Managing Organizational Conflict (Englewood Cliffs, NJ: Prentice-Hall, 1974), pp. 12–14.
4. J. Hall & M. S. Williams, "A Comparison of Decision-Making Performance in Established and Ad Hoc Groups," Journal of Personality and Social Psychology, 1966, 3, pp. 214–222.
5. Robbins, op. cit., Managing Organizational Conflict, pp. 12–14.
6. K. W. Thomas, "Conflict and Conflict Management," in M. D. Dunnette (ed.) Handbook of Industrial and Organizational Psychology (Chicago, IL: Rand McNally, 1976) p. 891.
7. L. Festinger, A Theory of Cognitive Dissonance (Evanston, IL: Row, Peterson, 1957).
8. R. A. Cosier and T. L. Ruble, "Research on Conflict-handling Behavior: An Experimental Approach," Academy of Management Journal, 24, 1981, pp. 816–831.
9. A. C. Filley, Interpersonal Conflict Resolution (Glenview, IL: Scott, Foresman, 1975), p. 52.
10. R. J. Burke, "Methods of Resolving Superior-Subordinate Conflict: The Constructive Use of Subordinate Differences and Disagreement," Organizational Behavior and Human Performance, 5, (1970), pp. 393–411.
11. H. Guetzkow and J. Gyr, "An Analysis of Conflict in Decision-making Groups," Human Relations, 7, (1954), pp. 367–381.
12. L. R. Pondy, "Organizational Conflict: Concept and Models," Administrative Science Quarterly, 12 (1967), pp. 296–320.
13. J. D. Aram & P. F. Jalispante, Jr., "An Evaluation of Organizational Due Process in the Resolution of Employee/Employer Conflict," Academic of Management Review, 6, (1981), pp. 197–204.
14. M. Dalton, "Conflict Between Staff and Line Managerial Officers," American Sociological Review, 15, (1066), pp. 3–5.
15. Daniel Katz and Robert L. Kahn, The Social Psychology of Organizations, 2nd ed. (New York: Wiley, 1978). See also Robert L. Kahn, D.M. Wolfe, R.P. Quinn, J. D. Snock, and R. A. Rosenthal, Organizational Stress: Studies in Role Conflict and Ambiguity (New York: Wiley, 1964) and

Andrew J. DuBrin, Fundamentals of Organizational Behavior: An Applied Perspective, 2nd ed. (Elmsford, NY: Pergamon Press, 1978).

16. Francine Hall and Douglas Hall, The Two-Career Couple (Reading, MA: Addison-Wesley, 1978).

17. National Association of Free-Standing Emergency Centers Report (1983).

18. R. T. Golembieski and A. Blumberg, "Confrontation as a Training Design in Complex Organizations," Journal of Applied Behavioral Science (October 1967), pp. 525–547.

Chapter Nine

HUMAN RESOURCES MANAGEMENT

A health care organization's ultimate success, whether it be a hospital or a small private practice, depends on how well the supervisor develops and maintains all of the human resources. The managerial function of staffing a department or practice is concerned with the development and maintenance of the organization's human resources to fulfill the institution's plans, objectives, and goals. For any health care organization the most important resource is its people. Other resources such as capital, the facility, and patient treatment equipment are essential to providing medical care. It is, however, the human element which determines the quality of health care delivered to the patient.

As a health care supervisor it is your responsibility to visualize the department's human resource needs and to staff it properly. The supervisor must carefully select employees and place them in positions which they are capable of handling. This is an important managerial respon—sibility. If an employee's capabilities do not match the requirements of the job, the individual will not derive satisfaction from its performance.

In the modern health care organization the staffing process includes a number of managerial activities. These activities include the selection, proper placement, development, training, and financial compensation of members of the organization. The health care manager is also charged with the responsibility of evaluating the performance of his or her employees. As such, the supervisor promotes employees based upon their efforts and abilities and rewards performance. The supervisor also has the ultimate responsibility of determining the manner by which to discipline improper employee behavior or, when necessary, discharge them from employment. Only when the health care manager fully understands as well as performs each of these vital functions can it be said that he or she is truly fulfilling the managerial staffing function.

THE ROLE OF THE PERSONNEL
DEPARTMENT IN THE HEALTH CARE INSTITUTION

In large health care organizations the personnel department (often referred to as the human resources management department) is actively involved in providing assistance and advice to managers at all levels in the organization. The personnel department's overall usefullness and effectiveness depends largely upon its ability to develop a good working relationship with department supervisors. To be an effective director of a physical therapy department, the supervisor must take full advantage of the expert advice, assistance, and services which are available from the personnel department.

The department of physical therapy and the personnel department must actively work together in all matters concerning the acquisition, training, promotion, discipline, and discharge of employees. As a health care supervisor, your primary role is to ensure that all patients receive high-quality care. To perform this function, the manager must make decisions concerning the qualifications required of employees who are to fill the staff positions. The supervisor is, therefore, responsible for determining in advance what is to be expected from new employees and provide the personnel department with the necessary information to assist in locating qualified applicants.

When a decision is made to acquire a new employee it is the personnel department's responsibility to contact the available market of qualified individuals who can effectively fill the position. As such, the personnel department accepts the responsibility for seeking out and attracting individuals to the organization. Quite often, the personnel department does this by contacting schools, colleges, professional associations, or professional recruiters who can provide assistance in creating the image of the hospital as an employer.

In most health care settings it is the personnel department who is responsible for conducting the preliminary interviews of all applicants for a position. The preliminary interviews are designed to ascertain if the applicant meets the necessary qualifications as outlined by the supervisor of the physical therapy department. It is the personnel department's responsibility to check professional qualifications and all references provided by the applicant. The personnel department should eliminate from consideration those applicants who do not meet the necessary criteria. Once the personnel department has determined those individuals who are eligible for employment, the department supervisor should then conduct his or her own interview.

Once the supervisor has met with all of the available applicants, the selection of the most qualified individual should be made. In some instances several interviews of the same applicant may be necessary depending on the importance of the position to be filled. The department supervisor, not the personnel department, should take final responsibility for hiring the individual. This is a role which should not be delegated to others. The supervisor should be the one to introduce the employee to the new job and assist in developing the person's skills and abilities.

The personnel department will take the initiative to introduce the new employee to the basic rules, procedures, and methods of operation which exist in the organization. The personnel department will also schedule any health-related tests which are required for employment. The director of the physical therapy department will, however, be responsible for introducing the employee to the physical requirements of the job, the wage system, the evacuation plans, as well as any other departmental information necessary for effective job performance. The personnel department will maintain records on the status of employment of each employee within the health care institution. This relieves the department director from a very burdensome task. Keeping a detailed record of each employee's date hired, promotions, salary history, vacation periods, disciplinary actions, and leaves of absence can be very complicated. This is especially true with the increasing numbers of pension programs and benefit plans within the modern organization. If the personnel department did not perform these tasks, they would greatly detract from the supervisor's ability to interact with department employees. As a result, most health care supervisors are delighted when the personnel department will take on these responsibilities and provide them with more time to interact with patients and employees.

One of the many benefits of the personnel department is the expert advice that can be provided. Advice is often needed because of the wide variety of personnel problems a supervisor may encounter. When the personnel department offers advice, guidance, or information, it will be done in a manner that assists the department director in making decisions.

A department director occasionally has difficulty in determining whether the personnel department is giving advice or attempting to make the decision. This can sometimes create tension between the two departments. To illustrate how advice and guidance differ from the personnel department's attempt to make the decision, consider the following situation:

> A physical therapist applies for a staff position at a hospital and requests special working hours other than those which are provided by the organization. Ideally, the personnel department should inform the department director of the applicant's request and advise the director of the possible personnel problems which can be created by making unusual accommodations for new employees. If, on the other hand, the personnel department rejects the applicant without notifying the department director, then no advice or information has been relayed.

The second situation, rejecting the applicant, is not inherently wrong on the part of the personnel department. Situations such as these may arise, not due to the personnel department's desire to broaden their authority, but rather as a result of the department's willingness to help prevent unwanted employment situations.

In most cases the director of physical therapy will welcome the personnel department's assistance in decision making. The physical therapist should realize that he or she has only a limited opportunity to visualize and appreciate the situation. For the organization to function smoothly, the department of physical therapy and the personnel department must work together in all personnel matters. Conflict situations can be avoided through joint cooperation.

Concerning the subject of decision making, the supervisor should allow the personnel department to make some of the decisions but certainly not all of them. When the physical therapy department encounters problems it is quite easy for the supervisor to blame the personnel department for unwanted consequences. If, for example, the department director receives a request from an employee for a raise, the easy solution is to simply state that, "Ordinarily, the raise would be possible, but the personnel department is not in a position to grant raises at this time." This temporarily clears the supervisor of the unwanted responsibility but will eventually lead to an erosion of authority. The supervisor will eventually appear as only a department figurehead. When encountering situations such as these, it is much better to state the truth and simply refuse to grant the raise.

The director of the department is also the individual who is in the best position to determine whether an employee should be discharged from the organization. In some instances, the personnel department may disagree with the department director's recommendation and advise the retention of the employee. If the employee is retained and the individual's performance remains unchanged or further deteriorates the supervisor is likely to develop an attitude of, "I told you so." There is also a chance the supervisor will avoid claiming any responsibility for outcomes which occur in the future. This reaction may be quite normal, but in the final analysis, it is the supervisor's responsibility for all events which transpire in the department. When placed in a position such as this the supervisor must continue to request the personnel department follow through on earlier recommendations.

In organizations where the personnel department does have final authority for discharging an employee it is often a power which has been granted by the top administrator. The top administrator has removed a part of the supervisor's authority and placed it in the hands of the personnel department. When this occurs, it may be the administrator's attempt to ensure guidelines are followed for proper termination of employees. Unfortunately, policies and procedures such as these may serve to erode the supervisor's position of authority in the eyes of subordinates. When policies such as these exist, the director of personnel should inform all department supervisors so as to prevent embarrassing situations when attempting to discharge an unwanted employee.

The physical therapist, in a supervisory position, should be continually updated on changes in government provisions regarding fair employment practices. All health care managers should be aware of how important it is to maintain proper employment documentation and how to avoid either conscious or unconscious discriminatory practices. The Civil Rights Act of 1964, Section 703A, Title VII states that:[1]

It shall be unlawful employment practice for an employer; (a) to fail or refuse to hire or to discharge any individual or otherwise to discriminate against any individual with respect to his compensation, terms, conditions, or privileges of employment because of such individual's race, color, religion, sex, or national origin; or (b) to limit, segregate, or classify his employees in any way which would deprive, to tend to deprive any individual of employment opportunities or otherwise inadvertently affect his status as an employee because of such individual's race, color, religion, sex, or national origin.

If the health care supervisor is unfamiliar with proper discharge practices or has not had the opportunity to participate in such action it may be advantageous to seek the opinion of the personnel department before initiating any discharge action.

PERFORMING THE MANAGERIAL STAFFING FUNCTION

In the health care organization the staffing function focuses on the managerial activities that deal directly with obtaining and developing human resources. Identifying, locating and hiring qualified health care employees is a continuous process. To properly perform the staffing function, the supervisor must recognize it as an ongoing activity which will change as individual members enter and leave the organization. The staffing function is sometimes mistakenly considered as only part of a new organization's attempts to fill employment positions. Regardless of the age of the organization, after awhile some employees will leave choosing to seek employment elsewhere. When this occurs it may call for an updating or changing of written policies and procedures to accommodate the requirements of new employees. It is, therefore, the health care supervisor's responsibility to ensure all matters concerning policies, procedures, and methods of organization remain applicable and that there is an adequate supply of qualified individuals to fill vacant positions.

ASSESSING EMPLOYEE REQUIREMENTS

The first step in assessing the number and type of employees needed for a health care organization is to evaluate the organization's present and future objectives and goals. At the department level, this is accomplished by examining present services and developing realistic expectations of additional services which could be offered in the future. For example, many hospitals have altered some of the services they offer as a result of the introduction of Medicare guidelines concerning diagnostic-related groups (DRG's). The implementation of these guidelines require hospitals to provide services in a specified manner if they are to be federally reimbursed.

As a result of these guidelines, hospitals are attempting to offer more comprehensive outpatient services. To be effective, the supervisor must carefully examine the organization's present design, anticipate the future, and plan the expansion of a department based on projected needs. Only by carefully studying the present design and direction of the organization can the supervisor anticipate future employment requirements. Deciding the type of jobs needed in a department and the qualifications of those who are to fill the positions is called job analysis.

Job analysis identifies what people do in their jobs and what they need in order to do the job satisfactorily. The purpose of job analysis is to collect information on the characteristics of a job that differentiate it from other jobs. Some of the information which must be gathered includes:

- The type of work to be performed.
- Working conditions that will be provided.
- Level of performance expected.
- Employee behaviors required.
- Equipment to be utilized.
- Supervision provided.
- The level of interaction with fellow health care professionals.

Job analysis outlines the demands to be made on the employee. The analysis should provide a description of acceptable performance and help to identify the type of person that should be considered for the job. As such, job analysis is the basis from which job descriptions and job specifications are developed and employee evaluations are performed.

DEVELOPING JOB DESCRIPTIONS AND JOB SPECIFICATIONS

Once the supervisor has decided on the type of employment position to be offered by the health care organization the next step is to outline the responsibilities of the jobs and the credentials required of those who are to fill the positions. To do so the supervisor must develop job descriptions. A job description is a written statement which carefully outlines the duties and requirements that are considered part of the job.

The objective of any job description is to outline every possible duty and responsibility that an employee is expected to perform. A written job description will establish performance standards. The performance standards will describe what the job accomplishes and what performance is considered satisfactory.

A job specification defines the qualifications of the person needed for the job. The job description describes the job, whereas the job specification lists the knowledge and skills needed to perform the job satisfactorily. As department supervisor it is your responsibility to determine the context of each position and the requirements of those individuals who are to fill the positions. Figure 9-1 is an example of a supervisory job description.

In situations where the supervisor is new to an established organization there should be written job descriptions already in place. One of the top priorities of a supervisor who is new to an established organization must be to become familiar with established policies. Through a careful review of established job descriptions the new supervisor can develop a better understanding of what tasks are required of the department's personnel. This allows the supervisor to understand the functions of present employees, why they do the things they do, and what should be changed. An occasional error of first-time supervisors is to make changes in an arbitrary fashion without first understanding why an employee does what he or she is doing.

When outlining the skills, abilities and educational requirements for a particular job, give careful consideration to exactly why you are asking for these qualifications. If an applicant becomes disgruntled after being rejected for a position of employment because he or she believes the "criteria are too stiff," the individual may accuse you and the organization of attempting to discriminate.

In one such case, the United States Supreme Court ruled that employment requirements must be job related.[2] In the *Griggs* vs. *Duke Power* case, the company maintained a promotion and transfer policy which required individuals to have both a high school diploma and to obtain a satisfactory score on two professionally developed aptitude tests. In one of the tests, blacks failed at a higher rate than whites.

In the decision, the Supreme Court established two points: (a) It is not enough to show lack of discriminatory intent if the selection tool results in a disproportionate effect that discriminates against one group more than another or continues a past pattern of discrimination; and (b) the

JOB DESCRIPTION

JOB TITLE: Director of Physical Therapy
DEPARTMENT: Physical Therapy

POSITION OF IMMEDIATE SUPERVISOR: Vice President, Chief Executive Officer.

I.   General Summary of Job Responsibilities: The director of physical
     therapy is responsible for the supervision of the staff, preparation
     of employee work schedules, participation in conferences, public
     education, public relations, assisting in patient treatment, and
     promoting professional growth. The director also prepares reports,
     the department budget, and any other related duties as required.

II. Specific Job Responsibilities:

     1) Preparation of schedules related to patient treatment,
         staffing, and statistical records.

     2) Guidance of personnel in goal attainment.

     3) Supervision of treatment procedures.

     4) Providing information to the public regarding the profession
         of physical therapy.

     5) Preparation of training programs for new personnel.

     6) Assist in administering patient care.

     7) Attendance at professional association meetings and conferences.

III. Job Specifications:

     Graduation from an accredited school of physical therapy with a bachelor
     degree in physical therapy. A masters degree in health related field
     is desirable. Five to ten years of progressive administrative experience.
     Ability to encourage people and establish support for programs and
     evaluate performance through established criteria.

Figure 9-1.

employer has the burden of proving that an employment requirement is
directly job related.

In this case the Supreme Court held that the intelligence test and the
high school diploma were not job related. For the supervisor it is important to remember that specifying a level of education or a long period of
experience is not necessary if all that is required is a short period of
training which can be performed after the individual is hired.

In general, the higher the director of physical therapy sets employment requirements, the more difficult it will be to find a person qualified
to fill the job. When establishing high job requirements be sure the job
will be a challenge to the person who eventually occupies the position. If
it is not, the new employee will soon realize that his or her abilities are

not being utilized to the fullest. This can create a situation where the employee rapidly becomes dissatisfied with the organization and resigns. This is not to say, however, that the supervisor should establish low employment standards. To define criteria too low will only result in a continuous stream of individuals that are unable to supply the quality of labor needed to provide patient care.

Understandably, the development of job descriptions and job specifications can be a lengthy process. The process can be shortened with the assistance of the personnel department. The personnel department may be of assistance in developing guidelines which are important to the organization. Once the job descriptions and specifications are near completion, the personnel department should review their content and make necessary recommendations. When the job description is in final form the personnel department should be provided with a copy to maintain in the department. This can be of assistance to the personnel department during the initial screenings of all job applicants. Following the outline of the job description the personnel department can compare prospective applicants with job requirements and refer only those qualified to the department supervisor for final acceptance or rejection.

It is the physical therapy supervisor's responsibility to review the contents of all job descriptions on a periodic basis. The knowledge required by the physical therapy employee, as well as the abilities needed to perform many of the health care services, are changing due to increasing technology and advances in science. When necessary, the supervisor should review and rewrite job descriptions. Periodic review is a requirement, since it is the job description that the personnel department refers to when interviewing a candidate. Without a periodic review and adjustment of the job description, there is an increasing chance of unintentionally selecting unqualified personnel to meet the changing demands of the health care organization.

THE INTERVIEW PROCESS

Once the director of physical therapy has developed job descriptions and job specifications, the next step in selecting a new employee will be the responsibility of the personnel department. The personnel department will perform the function of recruiting and narrowing the field of qualified health care professionals for a position within the health care organization. When this has been completed, it is then the supervisor's responsibility to interview each candidate and select the one most qualified. The interview can be a difficult process for both the supervisor and the prospective employee. The supervisor must evaluate each candidate's abilities and attempt to match them with the demands of the job. The supervisor additionally must determine whether the potential employee can handle the various responsibilities, working conditions, and demands the job has to offer. Determining these important factors can be difficult, since most employee interviews last only a few moments. In order to be successful in selecting and retaining employees for a department, the supervisor must have a thorough understanding of the types of interviews which may be conducted and their importance to employee morale and satisfaction.

There are primarily five types of interviews the physical therapy supervisor will encounter. The first of these is the pre-employment interview. In the pre-employment interview, the supervisor questions the candidate about his or her qualifications and interests concerning the employment position. Second, there are counseling sessions where the supervisor makes time available to discuss problems, sometimes personal in nature, which the employee is having. Third, there are termination interviews which discuss why an employee is being released from the organization. Fourth are the interviews which discuss why an employee is voluntarily leaving the organization. Lastly, there are those interviews which are conducted to review the employee's performance appraisal. For purposes of this text the five types of interviews will be grouped into two categories: those which are directive and those which are non-directive. It should be noted, however, that many of these interviews contain characteristics of both categories and can, therefore, be difficult to classify with absolute certainty.

The Directive Interview

The pre-employment interview is one of the most frequently cited examples of a directive type of interview. The primary purpose of a directive employee interview is to obtain enough information to make an informed decision about a prospective employee. In an interview such as this, the supervisor has a specially prepared group of questions which must be asked of each candidate. To ask these questions, the supervisor must set aside sufficient time to properly prepare for the interview. No prospective employee can be effectively evaluated unless the supervisor has taken sufficient time to review all available background information.

To prepare for the interview the supervisor should first request all information the personnel department has obtained concerning the background of the individual. The supervisor may discover the personnel department has obtained information which warrants direct discussion during the interview. The application blank, for example, may provide important information about an individual which cannot be obtained from a resumé. Having each prospective employee fill out an application blank provides subtle clues about personality and attention to detail. An application blank which is completed in a haphazard manner, with little or no regard to punctuation or spelling, may indicate future personnel problems.

When studying the application blank the supervisor should note any large time periods of unemployment or frequent changes in jobs. Where certain areas of employment appear questionable, the supervisor should discuss them during the interview. The techniques used by the supervisor do significantly affect the quality of information obtained. Some interview recommendations include:

1) USE OPEN-ENDED QUESTIONS. The use of open-ended questions helps prevent yes and no answers. Beginning questions with who, what, when, how, why, and tell me will generally produce more informative answers. "What is your approach to rehabilitation of a total knee replacement" is a better question than "Do you like working with patients who have had a total joint replacements?" The latter question will generally be answered yes or no.

2) AVOID LEADING QUESTIONS. A question is considered leading when it is obvious what the correct answer is simply by the way in which the question was asked. For example, "You like working with patients who present a wide variety of diagnosises, don't you?" For someone highly interested in the position the answer will probably be, "Of course."

3) DON'T ASK ILLEGAL QUESTIONS. Illegal questions are those which ask an individual's race, creed, national origin, marital status, number of children, and age. Asking questions concerning where the individual attends church or what political party they belong to are not job related. If, however, the person indicates they do

have children, it is appropriate to ask if arrangements have been made for child care during normal working hours.

4) ASK JOB-RELATED QUESTIONS. An interviewer who asks questions about what activities an applicant likes to engage in outside the job often does so in an attempt to "break the ice." The idea behind questions of this type is to help the candidate relax and feel more comfortable with the organization. In most cases, the prospective employee will not relax when it is apparent the supervisor is only making idle conversation. Questions of this type are also common when the supervisor is unprepared and using the time during the candidate's response to review the application form or resumé.

Additional Considerations

The supervisor should provide the personnel department with the most appropriate times to conduct interviews. An employment interview should not be conducted when the supervisor is rushed or the department is busy. Always attempt to conduct the major portion of the interview in the privacy of an office. Interviews should not be conducted in front of present employees where the conversation between the supervisor and the applicant can be overheard. If the physical therapy department does not have a quiet area for interviewing, request the personnel department provide an office. In all cases, avoid as many interruptions as possible. The supervisor should not leave an impression of being distracted or preoccupied with other matters. Remember, the prospective employee is also interviewing the supervisor. The impression you make will influence the employee's eventual decision concerning the attractiveness of the working environment.

Throughout the interview process try to put the applicant at ease. Every applicant is a stranger to both the organization and to its members. The applicant may be nervous while attempting to provide the best answers to questions. No interview should begin with an immediate discussion of the organization and the demands of the job. Instead, ask the prospective employee about their impressions of the local community. It is during this time you should assist the person in feeling at ease. Discussing the local community, prospective housing, and what the community has for entertainment and recreation are ways to introduce the person to the area in which the organization is located.

Besides obtaining information from the applicant the supervisor should also provide the opportunity for the individual to get to know the organization. The supervisor should be honest about the advantages and disadvantages of the department and the organization. Included should be a discussion of the salary, working hours, benefits, and periods of vacation. If the individual is a physical therapist or physical therapy assistant, the supervisor should discuss the health care organization's willingness to reimburse for professional dues and attendance at state or national professional association meetings. Additionally, the supervisor should indicate who will be the candidate's immediate supervisor. Overstating the potential satisfaction from a job or the likely benefits to be derived can lead to problems after the individual is hired and discovers the realities of the position. The employee who finds a job to be just as described in the interview will have greater respect and confidence in the supervisor and the health care organization.

Remaining Objective About the Applicant

One of the primary problems encountered in pre-employment interviews is for the supervisor to remain objective about the applicant. Factors such as the applicant's educational background and employment history are relevant, but the supervisor's personal preferences and prejudices are not. Many interviewers form an impression too early and spend the balance of the interview looking for evidence to support their ideas or beliefs. Research indicates that interviewers frequently make a decision on an applicant within the first four or five minutes. Making a decision about high-quality applicants usually takes longer.[3] To remain objective throughout the interview process requires an understanding of the potential areas where the supervisor will most often deviate.

One problem commonly encountered is the "halo effect." Here, the interviewer allows some very prominent characteristic to overshadow other evidence. An applicant may, for example, dress well and have an attractive physical appearance. The supervisor may base his or her employment decision on the belief that because the person is neat in appearance they will also be diligent in performing their job. After the individual is hired, job performance may not prove this to be the case. The "halo effect" can work either in a positive or negative fashion, but for purposes of employee selection it would be risky for the supervisor to form an opinion concerning an applicant based on the identification of a single factor.

Another problem with objectivity develops when the supervisor mistakenly compares the applicant and his or her qualifications with those of other members in the health care organization. For example, an applicant may be shy and reserved which is in sharp contrast to the personality characteristics of other employees. As a result of this outward personality difference, the supervisor may believe the person is unlikely to become an asset to the organization. The supervisor who follows this philosophy may overlook a health care professional who could greatly contribute to patient care and to the health care organization.

Lastly, studies have shown that unfavorable information greatly affects decisions concerning overall suitability. If information about an applicant is unfavorable, it may be given twice as much weight as favorable information. A single negative characteristic may bar the individual from being accepted, while no amount of positive characteristics will ensure an applicant's acceptance.[4]

The Results of the Interview

Once the supervisor has completed the interview he or she is then presented with three options: to reject the applicant, to hire the individual, or to postpone a final decision until a later date. If the applicant is found to be employable, announcing the decision to the person should be straightforward. All that remains is to establish a date to begin work. If, however, there are several applicants to be considered the supervisor may delay making a final decision until all have been interviewed.

When the supervisor has several applicants to interview, each candidate should be advised of the approximate time period which will lapse before a decision is to be made. If, however, the applicant has little or no chance of being considered for the position, the supervisor should not use a lengthy time period to avoid telling the individual the truth. Informing the person that he or she is unacceptable can be a difficult task. Despite the difficulty, it is only fair to advise the person of your decision so they can pursue other employment opportunities. To allow the person to wait an extended period of time may deny them the opportunity to obtain employment elsewhere.

When informing an applicant that he or she is not qualified for employment, do so in a polite and courteous manner. Try to provide the person with encouragement about the positive characteristics and abilities they possess which will be of value to them in the future. A standard turn-down phrase such as "In my opinion, we do not have a match between your qualifications and the needs of the organization. Unfortunately, this is likely to result in not using your qualifications to their best advantage" is considered appropriate. Giving specific reasons for not hiring encourages potential arguments and provides an opportunity for the supervisor to be misquoted.

Immediately after the interview the supervisor should record in writing the reasons why the applicant should not be hired. In rare instances a disgruntled applicant may imply that the interview and subsequent denial of a job was biased. Recording the reasons for a decision will help to refresh the supervisor's thinking. Written recordings are especially important if there are a large number of applicants applying for one position.

When conducting an employment interview the physical therapist must remember there are two organizations being represented. The supervisor is in a position to build a good reputation for both the profession of physical therapy and the health care organization. In many cases, the only contact the prospective employee will have with either the profession or the health care organization will be through the interview process. It is, therefore, essential the interview process be one which leaves a good impression with the prospective employee. Even though every person will not be hired, each individual should leave the interview with the feeling of having been offered a fair deal in a courteous manner.

Non-Directive Employee Interviews: An Integral Part of the Manager's Job

The non-directive interview, sometimes referred to as the counseling interview, presents a situation where the health care manager is interested in learning how an individual employee feels about a specific topic. The non-directive interview is frequently used when the employee wishes to discuss a specific complaint or as part of the exit interview when the individual is leaving the job.

The non-directive interview can provide a vital function for the health care organization. The interview provides the employee with an opportunity to express both feelings and ideas which may help to shed light on greater problems within the organization. Throughout these interviews, the employee should be encouraged to express his or her honest opinions without fear of reprisal. Whenever employees believe they cannot openly express their opinions, damage will result to the morale of the department.

Since the primary objective of the non-directive interview is to allow the employee to fully express problems, ideas, or attitudes, the interview must be conducted with caution. To properly conduct a non-directive interview requires the continuous attention of the supervisor. The supervisor must listen carefully to what is being stated or implied while exerting, at times, a considerable amount of self-control. In all cases the supervisor should avoid expressing emotion or indicating any approval or disapproval concerning the subject matter.

Many times, the counseling interview will serve the sole purpose of letting the employee express emotion. Some emotions will have been withheld for long periods of time. Once verbalized, the employee often expresses relief and may in the course of the discussion have discovered the source of the problem and developed a potential solution.

When conducting either a counseling interview or discussing why an employee is leaving the organization it is essential the supervisor allow the conversation to proceed with as few interruptions as possible. The supervisor should not attempt to answer phone calls or rectify other departmental matters. If the supervisor appears distracted it may leave the impression that he or she is disinterested or unconcerned.

Above all, the health care supervisor should avoid providing any advice or recommendations for an employee's personal problems. Quite often, the employee simply wants someone to listen, a sympathetic individual who can be trusted but refrains from offering advice. Offering potential solutions or becoming involved in an employee's personal matters will often extend beyond the organization and can meet with unintended consequences.

When presented with situations where an employee requests advice, do not hesitate to be straightforward and truthful about your reluctance to offer a solution. Tell the employee you are indeed sympathetic to the problem, but encourage them to seek the advice of someone trained in the area of concern. Throughout the next several weeks demonstrate continued interest in the employee, not the problem. Continue to be both supportive and encouraging. The health care supervisor who demonstrates a genuine interest in the well-being of fellow health care professionals will, in the long run, have significantly fewer personnel problems.

THE TERMINATION INTERVIEW

The termination of an employee is the most drastic form of disciplinary action. Termination of an employee will only be performed after a serious offense, such as stealing, or after having been repeatedly warned to cease an activity or an inappropriate behavior. For the health care supervisor the termination interview may be a difficult process, since it is ultimately the department supervisor's responsibility to provide the employee with specific reasons for dismissal.

All termination interviews should be conducted with the full knowledge and consent of the personnel department. The interview can be conducted very professionally by following a few simple steps.[5]

1) BE DIRECT. Tell the employee that, despite the effort on both sides, job performance has not been to your satisfaction.

2) INDICATE THE FINALITY OF THE DECISION. Any pleas for another chance should be disregarded.

3) REMAIN BRIEF. Meetings such as these should remain brief. Repeated discussions of weaknesses, already identified, may lead to employee anger and hostility.

4) EMPHASIZE GOOD POINTS. Soothing an ego can be beneficial. Reinforce the positive areas of an employee's work that can be taken to the next job.

5) TELL THE EMPLOYEE WHEN THE TERMINATION IS EFFECTIVE. In most instances the termination will be immediately effective. Unless there is a specific duty which must be completed, the employee should leave at the end of the interview.

6) GIVE SOME IDEA OF THE TYPE OF REFERENCE YOU WILL PROVIDE. Tell the person exactly what reason will be given for dismissal.

7) DISCUSS THE SEVERANCE PACKAGE. A severance package, sometimes referred to as the dismissal package, includes all monies owed to the employee. The package will include items such as salary, vacation, unused sick leave, and money in lieu of notice. The personnel department will take responsibility for preparing the package.

8) DISCUSS WHO SHOULD INFORM THE STAFF. This can be avoided if the dismissal is done at the end of the day. However, do not terminate an employee without having someone else present as a witness.

9) EXPRESS YOUR BEST WISHES IN FUTURE EMPLOYMENT OPPORTU-

NITIES. Try to end on a positive note. Thank the employee for his or her cooperation.

10) DOCUMENT AS MUCH OF THE CONVERSATION AS POSSIBLE. Include comments made by both parties.

Once terminated, the employee may react with anger towards you and the health care organization. Proper documentation for the specific reason of dismissal is important if age, sex, religion, race, or national origin can be implied as factors which influenced the termination decision. Additionally, the former employee may spread rumors about you and the organization. These should be of little concern, since most individuals will recognize the derogatory statements as coming from a disgruntled former employee.

THE APPRAISAL INTERVIEW

After the health care employee has been selected for a position and has worked at the job for awhile, the individual should have his or her performance reviewed. The appraisal interview is a special type of interview which provides feedback concerning performance. The interview is, to a large extent, a directive interview. It may, however, take on some of the non-directive aspects of the counseling interview.

The appraisal interview can be beneficial to the organization, the employee, and to the supervisor, if it is done properly. Many factors are identified in the performance appraisal including the employee's strengths and weaknesses, as well as those skills that are needed for the employee to develop and become eligible for pay raises and promotions. Due to the importance of the appraisal process the chapter which follows is devoted entirely to the managerial process of appraising a subordinate's performance and acting upon the results it provides.

REFERENCES

1. Civil Rights Act, 1964, Title VII, Section 703A.
2. Griggs vs. Duke Power Co., 401 U.S. 424 (1971).
3. William L. Tuller et al., "Effects of Interview Length and Applicant Quality on Interview Decision Time," Journal of Applied Psychology, 64, (1979), pp. 669–674.

4. T. W. Dobmeyer and M. D. Dunette, "Relative Importance of Three Content Dimensions in Overall Suitability Ratings of Job Applicant Resumes," Journal of Applied Psychology, 54, (1970), p. 69.

5. Mark A. Brimer, Fundamentals of Private Practice in Physical Therapy (Springfield, IL: Charles C Thomas, 1988), pp. 120–121.

Chapter Ten

APPRAISING EMPLOYEE PERFORMANCE

THE VALUE OF THE PERFORMANCE APPRAISAL
THE PERFORMANCE APPRAISAL PROCESS
SOME FACTORS INFLUENCING THE APPRAISAL OUTCOME
TYPES OF APPRAISAL
   Common Rating Scales
   Ranking and Forced Distribution
   Management by Objectives
      Advantages Of Management By Objectives
      Keys To Success In An M.B.O. Program
THE APPRAISAL INTERVIEW:
PROVIDING FEEDBACK ABOUT PERFORMANCE
PROMOTING AN EMPLOYEE
CRITERIA TO CONSIDER FOR PROMOTION
THE RIGHT COMBINATION

One of the most important functions performed by the health care supervisor is that of evaluating a staff member's performance. Beginning with the physical therapist's decision to accept a position within the organization and continuing through to their induction, training and counseling, the professional is growing in their knowledge about providing health care services. An important aspect of the development process is the performance appraisal. A performance appraisal serves to let the employee know of their value to the organization as well as indicating the possibility of promotion or additional compensation.

All health care organizations, regardless of size, evaluate or appraise employee performance in some fashion. In large health care institutions, such as a major medical center, the performance appraisal is likely to be a very formal procedure in which the performance of all managerial, professional, and clerical employees are assessed. As defined, the performance appraisal is a systematic means of determining how well an individual performed a job during a specified period of time. Additionally, it identifies what goals should be established in the future to correct or improve individual performance. The purpose of the performance appraisal is to further the development of an employee's career. Correctly viewed, it should be a positive encounter for the supervisor and for the staff member.

THE VALUE OF THE PERFORMANCE APPRAISAL

Unfortunately, the subject of performance appraisal is not always viewed in a positive way by the health care professional. The supervisor frequently dreads the prospect of appraising another's performance. Typically, the supervisor expresses embarrassment regarding the delicate nature of the process or has fear the employee may become angry and hostile if dissatisfied with the review process. Other supervisors see the purpose of the performance appraisal only as a tool for correcting unwanted performance and therefore resist the annual or semi-annual disturbance the process frequently creates.

Employees often express skepticism over the thought of being judged. When an employee is dissatisfied with the results of the appraisal, they frequently question the supervisor's ability to perform the appraisal or distrust the motives behind the process. Surprisingly, some employees see the appraisal process as beneficial, since it provides feedback concerning where they stand and how they can change behaviors in order to advance in the future. Others are indifferent to the entire process and plan to continue their tasks in the same manner regardless of how management views their performance.

Despite the wide variety of opinions supervisors and employees have about the performance appraisal, it is of value to the health care organization. Figure 10-1 and the following information outlines the importance.

TRAINING AND DEVELOPMENT, One of the most common uses for the performance appraisal is for training and development. Using the performance appraisal for training and development helps identify individual strengths and weaknesses. Once the supervisor has identified the positive and negative aspects of an individual's behavior and performance, steps can be taken to further increase skills and abilities and enhance performance.

FINANCIAL COMPENSATION. The appraisal can be used as a written justification for granting or denying employee pay raises. The performance appraisal will help to identify those employees who have performed above expected levels.

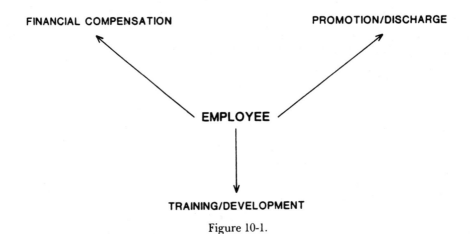

Figure 10-1.

PROMOTION OR DISCHARGE. The performance appraisal can be used as a basis for granting the employee a promotion or for discharging the individual from the organization. Those employees who have demonstrated skills and abilities worthy of promotion can be identified through the appraisal process. Employees who have not achieved supervisory expectations must also be identified through the appraisal process before being discharged from the organization.

Conducting the performance appraisal may be done in either an informal or systematic procedure. The informal appraisal is commonly performed by the supervisor on a daily basis. During an informal appraisal of performance the supervisor comments on various aspects of an employee's behavior as a means of providing feedback. The appraisal follows no established pattern and primarily exists as a conversation between the supervisor and the subordinate. The conversation may occur anyplace within the organization where work is performed.

The systematic appraisal is a formal process the supervisor and the health care organization use to evaluate performance. Most health care organizations conduct systematic appraisals on either an annual or semi-annual basis. The presence of a regular appraisal is important to employees in the health care setting. In large physical therapy departments, it is not uncommon for an employee to develop the feeling that he or she has been forgotten or lost. When the organization performs regular appraisals there is more assurance that an employee's contributions will be recognized and that management has an interest in the individual's performance.

THE PERFORMANCE APPRAISAL PROCESS

Most health care organizations have established methods by which to evaluate the performance of their employees. The personnel department will be responsible for designing an appraisal program and training the department supervisor in the proper methods of employee evaluation. The formalized system established by the personnel department will be used throughout the organization so as to allow all managers and department supervisors to speak the same language with one another and with the personnel department.

The process of appraising performance is generally recognized as proceeding through five steps. The appraisal process begins with the health care organization establishing a policy that a review process will be performed on an annual or semi-annual basis. Once the need has been identified, the second step is for the department supervisor to develop job descriptions, job specifications, objectives, and goals for each job.

After it has been established what aspects of employee performance are to be measured, the third step is to select an instrument to use in evaluation. There are a number of options available to evaluate the performance of an employee. Some of the most common and applicable to the health care environment will be discussed in subsequent sections of this chapter.

The fourth step in the evaluation process is one which must be performed exclusively by the health care supervisor. Evaluating a subordinate's performance is based on the assumption that the department manager is the most qualified individual to evaluate worker behavior and performance. The theory behind this approach is called the "unity of command." The unity of command principle is the belief that there is one person in each department who has the authority to make decisions. Each employee has a single immediate supervisor who is in turn responsible to his or her immediate supervisor. Following this concept allows everyone in the organization to know who their immediate supervisor is, where they stand, and who should and can give orders.

The final step in the performance appraisal process is that of interviewing the employee. For the supervisor and the employee the fifth step may be the most difficult. Interviewing the employee involves relaying the information which has been gathered. Here, the supervisor performs the important functions of offering praise, recognition, criticism, and providing suggestions about how performance can be improved.

As demonstrated in Figure 10-2, reviewing an employee's performance is the process of identifying, measuring, and developing human performance in the health care organization. The performance appraisal process must not only measure an employee's performance objectively but must also contain reinforcements which allow the employee to improve future performance.

STEP 1	STEP 2	STEP 3	STEP 4
Establish a policy to review performance	Develop job descriptions and set goals	Select an appraisal instrument	Evaluation by supervisor

STEP 5
Meet with the employee

Figure 10-2.

SOME FACTORS INFLUENCING THE APPRAISAL OUTCOME

The system of appraisal implemented in the modern health care organization must be designed to be as simplistic and straightforward as possible. It should not require an extensive mathematics background in order to compute an individual's final score. To prevent the implementation of complicated appraisal systems the personnel department should work in conjunction with the supervisor's suggestions as to what and how performance should be evaluated. Many of the uncomplicated appraisal forms include factors which adequately provide criteria for objectively measuring job performance. Some of these criteria include job knowledge, ability to carry out assignments, judgment, attitude, professionalism, adaptability, absenteeism, tardiness, and personal appearance.

Although unintentional, the supervisor is sometimes influenced by his or her like or dislike for a particular employee. Allowing personalities to influence the appraisal process is not fair to the employee. Supervisors who have experienced this problem often take corrective measures by simply evaluating several employees at the same time. The supervisor will perform the written evaluation of several employees rather than concentrating on just one. The intent of this method is to objectively compare performance without the injection of the supervisor's personal biases.

The supervisor should also remain aware of the "halo effect" in the performance evaluation process. Here, the supervisor rates an employee either high or low in one area of job performance and follows a similar pattern throughout the rest of the evaluation. The supervisor may, for example, strongly like one aspect of the individual's attitude and give the person high marks on everything else. The halo effect is different from simply liking or disliking an employee. When the halo effect is an issue, the supervisor may be so impressed (or unimpressed) with one aspect of an individual's behavior that he or she automatically assumes that everything else will be performed in the same manner.

The concept of "central tendency" is another problem the supervisor may encounter. Central tendency occurs when the supervisor simply goes down the evaluation form and rates the employee as only "fair" on all areas of job performance. Here, the supervisor does not want to recognize above average levels of performance but also wishes to avoid antagonizing the subordinate by rating the individual too low. The supervisor may dislike the evaluation process and only hopes not to anger anyone. One of the problems central tendency may create for the organization is that employees are rarely reinforced for excellent levels of performance and seldom advised of inappropriate behavior.

The supervisor should be careful to base the evaluation of performance on the entire period of time since the last appraisal. All behavior and job performance should be considered, not just instances when an employee did particularly good or bad. If the supervisor conducts the appraisal on an annual basis it is recommended to record incidents, both good and bad, that occur throughout the year. This helps the supervisor to recall specific events that are worthy of mention during the appraisal process. The supervisor should not, however, imply that he or she is maintaining a diary which can be used against employees at a later date. The purpose of documentation of this type is to enable the supervisor to provide employees with specific incidents which are examples of the quality of care the organization is looking for its members to provide.

As previously indicated, all employees should be evaluated by the individual to whom they report. Normally, the department director will assume the responsibility for evaluations performed in the department.

If the department has an assistant director, he or she may actively participate in the review process. Allowing the assistant director to participate in the review process serves two functions. First, and most importantly, it allows the assistant director to become familiar with the process of evaluating health care professionals fairly. Secondly, it provides the department director with additional information on which to base the evaluation. Without the assistant director's input the additional information may otherwise be unobtainable.

TYPES OF APPRAISAL

The appraisal of a health care employee's performance may be conducted using a number of different methods. The graphic rating scale, the frequency rating scale, and the forced-choice technique are all common category rating methods. The ranking and forced distribution techniques are additional methods for evaluating employee performance. Management by objectives is recognized as guided self-appraisal. The important characteristics of each will be discussed in the following.

Common Rating Techniques

One of the oldest and most common methods of evaluating a staff employee's performance is the rating scale. The evaluation of performance using the rating scale recognizes the existence of three types of scales: the graphic rating scale, the frequency rating scale, and the forced-choice technique.

The graphic rating scale will include a list of traits or characteristics that are considered important to job performance. Items to be considered for appraisal include: the quality of work, dependability, initiative, and cooperation. A specific number of points are assigned to each trait. The sum of the points becomes the total score for the individual being appraised.

The graphic rating scale allows the supervisor to judge an individual's existing talent for a particular trait. For example, the rating of dependability may be as follows:

Employee's Dependability

Extremely High	High	Medium	Low	Extremely Low
5	4	3	2	1

The supervisor will either circle or check the category which best describes the employee's behavior. Since the evaluation is based on the supervisor's opinion, it is important to recognize that individual biases and prejudices can be influential in the evaluation. Figure 10-3 is an example of a rating scale appraisal.

To appraise an employee's performance in present position, check ( ) the most appropriate square. The supervisor is encouraged to use freely the "REMARKS" section for recording significant comments descriptive of the individual.

1. KNOWLEDGE OF WORK:	Needs instruction or guidance.	Has required knowledge of own and related work.	Has exceptional knowledge of own and related work.
Remarks:			
2. INITIATIVE:	Lacks imagination.	Meets necessary requirements.	Unusually resourceful.
Remarks:			
3. APPLICATION:	Wastes time.	Steady and willing worker.	Exceptionally industrious.
Remarks:			
4. QUALITY OF WORK:	Needs improvement.	Regularly meets recognized standards.	Consistently maintains highest quality.
Remarks:			
5. VOLUME OF WORK:	Should be increased	Regularly meets recognized standards	Unusually high output.
Remarks:			

ADDITIONAL REMARKS:

Supervisor Signature	Date	Employee Signature	Date

Figure 10-3.

The frequency rating scale utilizes a quantitative choice rather than a description of performance. In appraising an employee's dependability the rating scale would appear as follows:

Employee's Dependability

Top   10%   20%   50%   20%   10%   Bottom

Obviously, the two rating scale methods may be prone to error. They often emphasize personality traits rather than objective measures of performance. One of the problems is that the terms used to describe the individual's performance will have different meanings to different supervisors. For example, words such as initiative may be interpreted differently when used in conjunction with words such as outstanding or poor.

The forced-choice technique requires the rater to check statements indicating what the employee is "most like" and another indicating what the employee is "least like." The statements appear in a mixed fashion presenting both positive and negative statements. It is the supervisor's responsibility to make the appropriate choices. When the appraisal is graded, usually by the personnel department, only one of the favorable items is given a positive credit and only one of the unfavorable items is given negative credit. Only those items which have a correlation or a relationship with efficiency will be utilized in determining the subordinate's performance. The purpose of implementing the forced-choice appraisal system is to reduce the rater's personal bias. An example of the forced-choice method is as follows;

Select statements below which most accurately or least accurately describe the employee. Place "M" (most) or "L" (least) in the space to the right.

1) Knows professional capabilities.   _____
2) Arrives to work on time.   _____
3) Does not document patient care.   _____
4) Demonstrates poor communication skills.   _____

Two of the characteristics are stated favorably: knows professional capabilities, and arrives to work on time. The other two characteristics— does not document patient care, and demonstrates poor communication skills—are stated unfavorably. When the appraisal is graded, item #1 will be given positive credit and item #3 will be given negative credit. They will be counted towards the performance appraisal. The other two, items #2 and #4, have less of a relationship with efficiency and job performance and will not be applied to the performance appraisal. Since the personnel department tabulates the results, the opportunity for the injection of personal bias is lessened, since the supervisor has no idea which of the items will be given credit.

Ranking and Forced Distribution

Ranking is the simple method of listing from highest to lowest the performance of all employees in a department. Utilizing this method, the supervisor would list each individual based on certain aspects of the worker's job or on the individual's overall performance.

One of the major drawbacks of the ranking method is that quite often there is little difference between those employees ranked close together. For example, employees ranked one, two, and three may be so close together in performance that it can be difficult to differentiate between them. Additionally, ranking means that someone will have to occupy the last position. This may result in morale problems for those ranked at or near the bottom.

The ranking process may be performed as follows:

Name of Employee

1. John Adams   6
2. Brenda Barnes   3
3. Sam Bigger   2
4. Richard James   4
5. Susan Johnson   5
6. Martha Smith   8
7. John Ubinger   1
8. Cindy Williams   7

All department employees are listed in alphabetical order to ensure no one is left out of the appraisal process. The supervisor would then rank those individuals considered as top performers, followed by those which are considered poor in job performance. The remainder would then be ranked somewhere in the middle.

Forced distribution is another method which ranks employees by class. Sometimes referred to as "grading on the curve," the method assumes the well-known "bell-shaped curve" of performance exists in a group. Utilizing this system of ranking assumes employees are representative of the total society. That is, some people may be rated high while others will be rated low. Figure 10-4 is an example of the type of scale used with forced distribution.

The forced distribution method can provide two serious drawbacks. First of all, the supervisor may resist placing individuals into the lowest group. Quite often it is difficult to explain to the employee why he or she was placed in one group while other similar employees were grouped much higher. Secondly, with small groups there is no reason to believe that a bell-shaped curve will exist. The curve may be skewed in one direction or the other.

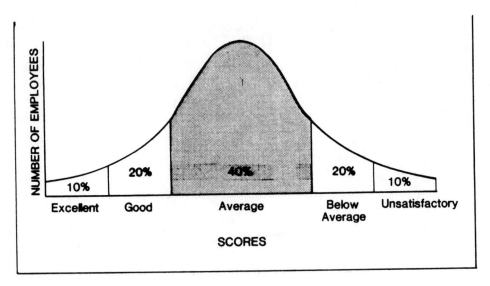

Figure 10-4.

Management by Objectives

Management by Objectives (MBO) is a managerial system that places considerable emphasis upon performance evaluation. First publicized by Peter Drucker in his book, *The Practice of Management,* and later by Douglas McGregor, management by objectives has become a popular approach to team management.[1] The technique has been adopted by some of this country's largest organizations and has met with considerable success.

The basis for the MBO process is the stronger an individual is committed to a goal, the more likely the person will work towards objective and goal accomplishment. The objectives and goals are established jointly by management and the worker. Once established, each is to be attained within a specified period of time. Management by objectives assumes that people like to be evaluated according to criteria they believe to be realistic and reasonably attainable. The supervisor is no longer a judge in the appraisal process but a coach who participates in setting goals and identifying the criteria that will be used to evaluate and reward performance. Some of the goals which are established are qualitative, such as "improved patient relations." Others, such as "increase in the volume of patients to be seen," are in quantitative terms.

To better visualize the MBO process, the supervisor must think of it in terms of six steps.

1) The manager and the subordinate review what the manager is to accomplish in the job. Here the manager discusses his or her role in the organization and what the organization must accomplish.
2) The manager and the subordinate discuss key components of the subordinate's job. The manager may review organizational job descriptions and job specifications with the subordinate.
3) The manager and the subordinate agree on objectives to be accomplished in a predetermined period of time. The time period usually does not exceed one year.
4) Throughout the time period the supervisor and the subordinate meet to discuss progress towards objectives. Periodically, the objectives may have to be modified to allow the subordinate to accomplish them.
5) Annually or semiannually the supervisor and the subordinate will meet to review the overall performance of the subordinate. This meeting will constitute the formal performance appraisal.
6) The supervisor and the subordinate will discuss the objectives and goals to be accomplished in the future. Once again, a time period will be established for accomplishment.

Advantages of Management by Objectives

Management by objectives offers three major advantages over the traditional rating systems. First of all, the supervisor and the subordinate identify objectives which are to be accomplished. The MBO process does not give subordinates a blanket privilege in setting their own objectives. Utilizing MBO emphasizes the "jointness" in objective development. The supervisor still retains final decision-making authority for approving objectives.

Second, specific end results are spelled out so that the level of performance is clearly identified. Clearly outlined goals and end results will facilitate the evaluation and reward processes. Properly developed objectives include such things as "to have employees attend a professional education seminar this year." A poor objective would be "to improve the quality of physical therapy offered by the department." Obviously, the first objective is measurable, whereas the second is far too broad to ascertain true accomplishment.

Third, by following the MBO approach, the worker and the supervisor establish future goals rather than utilizing other methods which simply evaluate the past. Management by objectives helps the manager and the subordinate plan for the future and conceptualize what it is their jobs are to accomplish. Both the manager and the subordinate identify the critical aspects of the job and direct their efforts toward achieving major performance targets.

Keys to Success in an MBO Program

1) Both the supervisor and the subordinate must establish clear and specific goals. Establishing goals which leave little or no room for speculation has a more positive effect on performance than simply indicating for the subordinate to do the best he or she can.

2) Establish difficult but attainable goals. Those goals which are perceived as too easy will present little, if any, challenge to the employee.

3) The supervisor should not simply assign goals. Performance can be improved through joint participation in goal development. As is seen in Figure 10-5, the supervisor and the subordinate must agree on what should be accomplished. The manager and the subordinate should use practice work sheets to formulate individual ideas before committing to a finalized form.

4) The supervisor must outwardly recognize, reinforce, and reward the subordinate's goal attainment.

5) All members of the organization must be committed to the MBO process. Commitment must come from top management's willingness to train supervisors and subordinates in the proper use of MBO.

6) There should not be an overemphasis on quantitative goals (dollars or the number of patients treated). Qualitative goals may be equally as important in the improvement of patient care.

To be effective, the MBO program requires a new system of interaction between the supervisor and the subordinate. The supervisor must move towards a more participative or "flexible" style of management. If the supervisor prefers an authoritarian style of management, he or she will need to be re-educated before the program can be successfully implemented.

SMITHTOWN HOSPITAL

Name _____

Department _____

- -

Performance rating: Excellent ☐   Very good ☐   Good ☐   Fair ☐
Unsatisfactory ☐   Very unsatisfactory ☐

- -

Job description

Achievements since last review

Goals

Career interest/development plans

Employee strengths/weaknesses

Replacements/position target

Supervisory signature

Employee signature

Figure 10-5.

THE APPRAISAL INTERVIEW:
PROVIDING FEEDBACK ABOUT PERFORMANCE

The final step in the appraisal process is for the supervisor to discuss the results with the employee. This may be the most difficult part, since no health care supervisor wants to create a situation which could lead to misunderstandings or even hostility. In all appraisal situations, it is imperative that the person who performs the evaluation of performance be the one who meets with the employee. No matter how difficult the interview process may be, the evaluation interview cannot be delegated to someone else.

Conducting an appraisal interview requires preparation. Prior to the interview the supervisor should review what areas of employee performance were assessed and be willing to indicate what results were expected. To ensure consistency, the supervisor should prepare a general outline to follow throughout the evaluation of all employees. The outline to follow should include each of the following:

1) PURPOSE OF THE EVALUATION. The supervisor should open with a brief statement to establish a rapport and encourage the subordinate to speak freely. Included in this statement should be an indication about how the evaluation was performed and the time period it covers. It is also acceptable to ask the employee how well he or she thinks the job was performed. Although unlikely, this provides the employee with an opportunity to self-criticize job performance.

2) REVIEW THE FINDINGS OF THE EVALUATION. Try to begin the review of performance by discussing the employee's strong points. If the employee did something noteworthy, recognize it and indicate its importance to the organization. Once the strong points have been discussed, the supervisor should review the weaknesses. When reviewing an employee's weaknesses, the supervisor should refrain from being too critical. State the problem areas clearly and in an objective fashion. Repeatedly emphasizing problem areas or inappropriate behavior may lead to employee hostility and resentment. There is certainly no established method by which to recognize achievement or provide criticism. Some health care supervisors believe it is best to start an evaluation interview with praise, then move to the critical points and end the interview on a pleasant note. The attempt here is to cushion the blow by providing good things at both ends of the interview. Unfortunately, the attempt to cushion the blow may not always be appropriate. The attempt by the supervisor to "downplay the negatives" may result in the worker forgetting about the criticism. The supervisor should always ap-

proach the interview by considering the individual as a mature adult capable of taking appropriate levels of criticism when it is provided in a respectful manner.

3) CLOSING THE INTERVIEW. No interview should be terminated with the two parties angry at one another. The supervisor should always strive to maintain self-control and encourage the subordinate to do the same. The appraisal interview is nothing more than a conversation between two health care professionals. Despite this fact, there will be times when the employee does not agree with the findings contained in the appraisal. When this occurs the supervisor must be prepared to cite how performance could have been improved. The supervisor should attempt to reach an amicable consensus. The goal still remains one of obtaining the subordinate's commitment to improving overall job performance.

The physical therapy supervisor sometimes feels as though the appraisal and interview process is unnecessary, since he or she is in continual contact with employees. This type of perspective can only lead to problems within a department. Every employee needs to know where they stand in the eyes of the organization. This can only be accomplished through a formal evaluation process where management and the employee openly discuss topics related to the job. Even though employees may not like the appraisal process any more than the supervisor, it is still a necessary and important part of health care supervision.

PROMOTING AN EMPLOYEE

One of the many benefits of conducting a performance evaluation is the identification of those employees who are worthy of a promotion. A promotion is a change in job assignment from a lower level job to a higher level job within the health care organization. Moving an employee to a higher level job usually means the employee will have to accept more responsibility but also generally provides an increase in pay and status.

The health care organization who adopts a policy of "promoting from within" can foster employee loyalty. Once employees recognize the health care organization adheres to the policy, the concept can act as an incentive for obtaining better work. When employees realize they can get ahead by knowing their job and remaining loyal to the organization, the work will often seem more challenging. Providing goals such as higher pay, better working conditions, and a sense of achievement can be powerful motivators. For the health care organization, promoting from within secures the services of an individual who essentially knows the organization better than any outside applicant possibly could. As a result, learning the new job and its responsibilities should be far less demanding and time consuming.

In some organizations, especially small hospitals, the policy of promoting from within is not always possible. When there are no qualified candidates the policy may meet with unintended results. As a supervisor, it is important to recognize that no employee should be placed in a position, especially managerial in nature, who has not had at least minimal exposure to health care supervision. Placing someone in a managerial position in hopes they can be trained or because they can be obtained for less cost than by recruiting from the outside is risky. The selection of the wrong person in a managerial position can rapidly deteriorate department morale.

In other instances, top management may recognize the need to obtain an individual with no previous ties to the organization. The idea behind this approach is that the new person will stimulate new ideas and methods of patient treatment. Administration will frequently make such changes when a long established supervisor leaves the organization. Top management may wish to dispose of the "dead wood," especially if there are plans to modernize the department. To implement plans of top management, a person with the necessary skills and abilities would be recruited to occupy the position. Some managerial positions, such as director of a burn unit, or director of a cardiac rehabilitation unit, may require extensive training in order to provide the necessary employee guidance and leadership. Only very large health care organizations can afford the time and expense of a lengthy training process. When presented with a deadline or lengthy and expensive training process, the organization may have no choice but to recruit from the outside.

It is important for the supervisor to recognize that not all employees are interested in a promotion opportunity. Some employees may look upon a promotion as requiring more time and effort than they are willing or able to assume. Others simply do not want to take on the added responsibilities which go with an increase in salary. It may also be possible that the employee likes the staff position because it provides more opportunity for patient care than would be allotted in a managerial position. Regardless of the employee's reasoning, the supervisor must recognize and respect the individual who is content in his or her present position and not pressure them into accepting an unwanted managerial position.

CRITERIA TO CONSIDER FOR PROMOTION

A health care organization which maintains a policy of attempting to promote from within hopes this will act as an incentive for employees to provide quality health care services. Those physical therapists and physical therapy assistants who demonstrate the necessary skills and abilities are the ones the organization believes should be promoted to positions of increasing job responsibility. When assessing an individual's ability to assume a job with greater responsibility, the supervisor should be aware of factors which may influence the decision-making process.

In many of the large industrial sectors of the United States, such as the automotive industry, labor unions have had a profound impact on which person is selected for promotion. Labor unions frequently encourage promotion based on seniority. Promoting an individual based solely on seniority limits the supervisor's choices, since it recognizes the person who has been with the organization the longest as the one who should be promoted. Although labor unions are not well established in the health care sector, many organizations use seniority as the basis for promotion if the employee has demonstrated sufficient training and ability.

Basing a promotion strictly on an employee's loyalty can pose a number of problems for the health care organization. In some instances, the person who has been with the organization the longest is not the best one to be placed in charge of a group of health care professionals. The assumption on management's part is that the individual's ability to supervise increases with the length of service. Unless the employee has been actively working and planning for the day when promoted to the position, it is unlikely the department will be enhanced by the selection. Relying solely on the length of service as a criteria for promotion is not an effective means of enhancing the growth of the department.

This is not to say, however, that relying to some degree on length of service is not a good idea. It does provide advantages to the organization. One advantage is ensuring that the employee chosen will be, at least to some degree, familiar with the job and the organization. Those health care organizations who stress seniority as crucial for promotion have often made a conscious effort to select employees who would someday be promotable. They have done this so they will always be in a position to place high-caliber people in strategic locations. Those physical therapists or physical therapy assistants who have demonstrated the necessary qualifications for promotion will be steadily increased in job responsibility.

Other factors which must be considered for promotion include the individual's professional skills and past performance. Professional skills are sometimes difficult to judge with certainty. Professional skills include those abilities to provide quality patient care and interact well with staff members, doctors, and members of top management. In evaluating past performance the supervisor must examine how the employee has performed in the past and project whether this behavior will be continued in the future. The supervisor should mentally place the individual in the job and estimate his or her level of performance.

THE RIGHT COMBINATION

In the modern health care organization no individual should be promoted strictly on the basis of one job-related factor. The decision for promotion should be based on a combination of factors which best suits the needs of the organization. When the final selection is made, the supervisor will frequently discover the person chosen is the one with the greatest length of service.

On the other hand, the final selection may be someone who has outstanding leadership ability and professional skills which far exceed the abilities of other applicants. The goal is, of course, to select the most qualified of applicants. Using criteria such as these provides the supervisor with a more complete look at the job to be filled and the person needed to occupy it. Not only are you assessing the person's loyalty but also their qualities as a professional and their record of consistent performance.

REFERENCES

1. Peter Drucker, The Practice of Management (New York: Harper & Brothers, 1954) and Douglas McGregor, "An Uneasy Look at Performance appraisal," Harvard Business Review, Vol. 35, No. 3, (May–June, 1957), pp. 89–94.

Chapter Eleven

HEALTH CARE BUDGETING AND FINANCE

B udgets are the most widely used forms of planning and control in the health care organization. Budgets are plans which express anticipated results in numerical terms. They are also an element of control, since they can be used to assess the actual progress toward the plan. Assessing progress toward the plan enables the supervisor to take action, whenever necessary, to make certain results conform to the plan. Top administrators and the board of directors are responsible for budget development for the entire organization. At the department level, each supervisor will be responsible for budget preparation.

Budgets may be expressed in terms of dollars, personnel hours, kilowatt hours, materials, or any other unit which is used to perform work. The most frequently used budget is the one which is expressed in monetary terms. The figures the supervisor puts into the budget are not mere projections or forecasts but will become the standards to be achieved. They will be considered the basis for daily operations and serve as an outline for goal accomplishment.

Budgets guide the supervisor throughout the period specified. The budget is an example of a single-use plan which will not be called upon again once the particular period is over. In order for the organization and its various departments to continue operation, a new planning period will be established and new budgets will be developed.

Every supervisor should participate in budget preparation. In order for budget development to be effective, it must be supported by members of top management. Middle and first level managers should be encouraged to submit timely budgets and substantiate their proposals in a discussion with the next level of management or the organization's top administrator. No budget should be submitted or accepted if it is based on plans which are inadequate or incorrect. Budgets should only be put into action when those who are responsible for executing them have a clear understanding of the allowances which are provided for goal accomplishment. Pseudo participation in budget development at any level in the organization will result in misunderstandings, miscommunications, and organizational ineffectiveness.

THE PROCESS OF BUDGETING

A budget is a written plan which serves as a blueprint for mapping the health care organization's future. Although the authority and responsibility for the budget ultimately rests with the administrator and board of directors of the institution, each supervisor should have a clear understanding of the budget's primary objectives. The objectives of a budget defined by the American Hospital Association are:[1]

1) The budget should provide a written expression, in quantitative terms, of the policies and plans of the hospital.
2) The budget should provide a basis for the evaluation of financial performance in accordance with established plans.
3) A budget should be a useful tool for the control of costs.
4) The budget should create an attitude of cost awareness throughout the organization.

The process of developing a budget for a large institution involves a number of individuals who perform varying roles within the organization. Each of these individuals or groups perform vital functions which enable the budget to be prepared and implemented. In large health care institutions, the following groups and individuals are generally involved:

- The Board of Directors
- The Chief Executive Officer
- Controller or Director of Finance
- Center Managers
- The Budgetary Committee

The board of directors are legally and morally responsible for the operation of the hospital. As has been attested to in repeated court actions and decisions, the ultimate responsibility for hospital operation and the level of care provided to the patient rests with the board of directors. The board of directors are responsible for determining policies, maintaining good community relations, maintaining professional standards, appointing and reviewing the activities of the medical staff, as well as ensuring adequate financing and control of expenses. The board helps in establishing the objectives and goals that are used in budget development. In most cases it is the board who formally approves the finalized budget.

The chief executive officer (CEO), or administrator, has the responsibility for implementing the policies and programs that have been delegated by the governing board. The administrator also has the responsibility of preparing a budget for approval by the governing board. The budget the chief executive officer prepares is an estimate of future expenditures. When the budget is approved by the board, it becomes the authority for the administrator to make expenditures.

Controllers serve the function of gathering relevant data on costs and outputs that may be used in budget development. Their responsibility is not in making or enforcing the budget but rather to be of assistance in providing data to support projected expenditures. In most health care institutions, those individuals in controller positions will have educational backgrounds in finance or be certified public accountants.

Center managers are the directors of the various departments within the health care institution. Each manager plays a role in determining how the health care institution will operate. Budgeting at the department level is often referred to as "grass roots" budgeting. Participation at this level is vital to the organization and a prerequisite for successful budget administration.

Some health care institutions establish a budgetary committee to aid in budget development. The committee is generally headed by the controller and has a membership consisting of several of the organization's top department heads. The committee does not take responsibility for preparing the budget but instead helps to legitimize the various budget estimates so that they do not appear arbitrary or capricious. Once completed, the final revisions will be given to the administrator for review. After final evaluation, the budget will then be submitted to the board.

The two most common ways to develop budgets are the top-down and bottom-up approaches. Although less common in the health care environment today, the top-down budget is an example of a budget which is almost exclusively developed by the members of executive management. Once the budget has been developed, it is then implemented at lower levels with little or no consultation. Those physical therapists new to health care management may find the organization will budget for their department until such time as they begin to feel comfortable with taking over the responsibility.

The bottom-up approach is a budgeting method in which department managers at each level are responsible for the development and implementation of their own department's budget. The bottom-up approach is more conducive to the modern view of health care management. Physical therapists are increasingly interested in setting the direction for department operation. Using the bottom-up approach provides the health care manager with the following advantages.

1) Physical therapists who are department directors are in a better position to evaluate the needs of their department. They know where cutbacks can be made and where additional funds should be allocated.

2) The important elements are less likely to be overlooked when utilizing the bottom-up approach. The supervisor can be more conceptual in predicting potential shortages and determining how they should be corrected.

3) Bottom-up budgeting gives the health care manager a sense of responsibility. The manager will be more motivated towards performance when the responsibility is shifted to the department level.

4) Evaluations of supervisor performance are much easier. Budgets provide immediate feedback concerning the director's ability to plan and control. The director of physical therapy who always exceeds budget projections is not as valuable to the organization as

one who can be relied upon to keep costs at or below projected levels.

Although the bottom-up approach is recognized as a more effective way of budgeting in the health care organization, it is not without its problems. The primary problem arises when managers overstate their requirements in order to secure adequate monies for their department. Actions such as these are done to ensure adequate self-protection. The manager wants to be on the safe side and estimates requirements high so as to stay within the allocated amount. The assumption is that if the manager can stay within the boundaries of the budget, he or she will be praised by top management. To discourage this type of behavior most administrators will indicate that they consider a number of factors in managerial evaluation other than simply budget compliance.

FORMULATING THE BUDGET

Every health care organization has a method it likes to follow when developing a budget. Budgets should be considered a tool for management and not a substitute for good judgment. Development of a budget must consider providing the supervisor with enough flexibility to properly accomplish departmental objectives and goals. Although most budgets are in numerical terms, the numbers should not be recognized as absolute or act as a limiting device in exercising good judgment and adaptability. To be effective, the manager should implement the following steps in bottom-up budgeting.

1) STATEMENT OF DEPARTMENTAL GOALS. The essence of the bottom-up approach to budgeting is that it allows managers flexibility in budget development. As such, the manager should state the necessary requirements as well as any realistic proposals. Included in this statement should be an economic forecast for the coming year as well as any new proposals that could improve the department's profit position. Avoid making any extraneous "wish lists." If you have physician support for the acquisition of new rehabilitation equipment, include that information in your statement. Obtaining the support of a medical staff helps expedite the purchase of new equipment.

2) ACTUAL BUDGET PREPARATION. The department manager has the ultimate responsibility for budget preparation. Budgeting should

never be postponed until the last moment. The department supervisor should plan throughout the year for ways to increase the efficiency and effectiveness of the department. Some of the best ideas submitted for budget consideration are those which are anticipated.

3) ADMINISTRATIVE REVIEW. Once the department director has completed the budget, it will be reviewed by the top administrator or by one of the vice-presidents. The department director must never assume that the administrator will automatically accept everything which has been proposed. The individual in charge of budget review may ask for supporting evidence for new proposals. Be prepared to defend and justify your requests.

4) BUDGET EVALUATION. Once the budget period has expired, the manager will be evaluated on his or her performance. Although the length of the budgeting period may vary from institution to institution, most are for a period of one year. New managers may have their budget performance evaluated on a quarterly or semi-annual basis.

In addition to annual budgets, hospitals may also have budgets that extend over a much longer period of time such as three, five, ten, or even as much as fifteen to twenty years in advance. These budgets, referred to as long-term budgets, usually cover such items as research or proposed expansion. Long-term budgets are developed by the chief executive officer and seldom concern the department supervisor.

TYPES OF BUDGETS

There are a number of budgeting methods available to the health care organization. This section introduces the health care professional to the basic terms associated with budgeting and discusses three important types. They are: the expense budget, the revenue budget, and the profit budget.

1) EXPENSE BUDGET. An expense budget details the future and projected costs for a specific responsibility, such as the department of physical therapy. Here, the financial concern is for the materials required, labor costs, and estimated overhead costs. When the health care manager exceeds the expense budget, it is an indication

that costs are higher than they should be and that a certain level of inefficiency exists.

2) REVENUE BUDGET. A revenue budget details the future and projected income for a specific center. In the department of physical therapy, the revenue budget would consist of the projected number of inpatients and outpatients which would be seen, the number of projected treatments, and their average cost to the patient. The revenue budget is understandably important to the organization but also highly uncertain, since it requires the manager to predict the future. To aid in forecasting the future, the manager may rely on historical data. It is important to recognize, however, that a revenue budget for a health care organization in a stable and uncompetitive environment will be more accurate than one developed for an unstable and competitive environment. Understanding the projected levels of change in an organization and community is vital for proper revenue budget development.

3) PROFIT BUDGET. A profit budget is the sum of the revenue and expense budgets. Profit budgets indicate whether individual departments will have control over their costs. Profits can, however, be misleading. There must always be a consideration as to whether or not the budgeted profit level was achieved according to the plan. No profit should be considered valid if it was obtained by resorting to cost-cutting efforts.

Throughout the budgeting process it is important to consider the fact that not all departments in a hospital will evidence an annual profit. Hospitals frequently have to offset the revenue obtained in one department against the losses acquired in another. Departments new to an organization will often be carried at a loss until medical doctors become aware of the services offered or until the surrounding community recognizes their health care value.

CONTEMPORARY BUDGETING APPROACHES

The budget is the formal expression of a plan used for setting objectives and for evaluating results. Although there are a wide variety of budgeting approaches available to the health care organization, all budgets have similar features. That is, there is a financial commitment by the organization, actual expenditures are computed, the variances from the projections are ascertained, and explanations for deviations are made. Among the most popular methods for profit and non-profit organizations are planning-programming-budgeting (PPB) and zero base budgeting (ZZB). Both are explained in the following sections.

Planning-Programming-Budgeting System

Developed during the Kennedy administration the planning-programming-budgeting system was first implemented by the Department of Defense. The system was initially introduced because previous budgetary systems had resulted in the armed forces duplicating a number of services and because other methods failed to provide for the long-term consequences of short-range budgetary decisions. The PPB system is in sharp contrast to the traditional one-year budgetary cycle. Funding under the PPB system is generally projected for three or more years. Since some programs take years to develop, the system is designed to allow enough time for the achievement of established long-term objectives and goals.

The PPB system was fully implemented under President Johnson in the late 1960s and subsequently abandoned in 1971.[2] The reasons for its lack of full implementation and acceptance were essentially due to improper instructions and procedures, as well as poor communication. Some agencies resisted it because they saw little benefit to be derived from it or because it was forced upon them without consultation.

Despite its lack of acceptance by those in federal government, the health care environment can benefit from understanding its methodology. The PPB system consists of five major steps:

1) The objective of each program is specified. Each department within the organization must determine what it is trying to accomplish. An all-out effort is made to make sure nothing is overlooked.

2) The present activities of each department are analyzed to determine if they promote the objectives and goals of the organization.

3) A program which is under consideration is evaluated in terms of long- and short-term costs. One-year costs are not considered as important as costs over the life of the program.

4) The organization considers all of the alternatives. Programs are compared to one another to determine which will be the most beneficial and cost effective.

5) The PPB system is integrated into the activities of each department within the organization. Success depends on organizational-wide implementation.

The primary disadvantage to the PPB system is that it is very time consuming. Long-range planning and the analysis of a program's cost effectiveness take considerable managerial effort. The process of reaching a final budget can be a costly endeavor in terms of the man-hours which must be committed. Additionally, commitment to and attainment of long-range objectives and goals can be especially difficult if personnel turnover is high.

Zero Base Budgeting

As the popularity of PPB system decreased, a new system of budgeting called zero base budgeting (ZBB) was introduced into many business organizations. Originally introduced at Texas Instruments, zero base budgeting gained national attention in the 1976 presidential campaign when Govenor Jimmy Carter announced he would implement it at the federal level if elected.[3]

Utilizing ZBB requires each department in the organization to annually develop a new budget. Prior to the introduction of ZBB, many managers would use the figures from the old budget to develop the new one. They assumed the figures in the old budget were correct and could be used to justify the new budget. Following the principles of ZBB, no such assumptions can be made. Zero base budgeting differs from the traditional methods of budgeting called "incrementalism." Traditional incremental budgets change each year only by modest increases or slight decreases. According to the ZBB method, a new budget must be developed from scratch (a zero base) with every dollar expenditure being justified. The budgeting system proceeds through three steps: the development of decision packages, ranking decision packages, and the allocation of resources.

1) THE DEVELOPMENT OF DECISION PACKAGES. The process of developing or formulating decision packages helps define a specific activity within an organizational unit. Included in the definition are the costs and benefits of each individual unit. Analyzing an activity or program provides management with relevant information concerning its costs and benefits to the organization. The

consequences of continuing or halting a program can be identified along with how other programs might be used to replace it.

2) THE RANKING OF DECISION PACKAGES. Once decision packages have been developed, the next step is to rank them in order of importance to the organization. The ranking of decision packages is performed by all managers, with a final ranking review by top management.

3) THE ALLOCATION OF RESOURCES. Resources are assigned to the organization's activities based upon the ranking received. Those activities ranked high receive more resources than those with lower ranks. Those activities which were ranked low may receive little or no funding at all.

Zero base budgeting offers both advantages and disadvantages. The primary advantage is that it forces the manager to scrutinize the effectiveness of all programs before ranking them. Those programs which are no longer beneficial to the patient, the organization, or considered cost effective can be eliminated. The disadvantage is that it also requires more time than the traditional methods of budgeting. The United States Navy tried zero balance budgeting and forwarded 2,000 pages of documentation to Congress rather than its customary 150 pages.[4]

SUCCESSFUL BUDGETING

The process of developing a budget should never become so time consuming that it becomes an exercise in frustration to those who must formulate and administer them. Excessive detail in budgeting, including the documentation of the smallest expenditure, demonstrates a weakness in the budgeting philosophy of the health care organization. Highly detailed budgets are time consuming and difficult to manage and live within. To develop and work effectively with budgets, managers should consider the following:

1) ALLOW LOWER LEVEL MANAGERS TO PARTICIPATE IN THE BUDGETING PROCESS. Top managers who develop budgets and simply present them to department supervisors often fail to gain an organizational-wide commitment. Managers at all levels can derive significant satisfaction from participating in the budgetary process.

2) BUDGETS SHOULD BE FLEXIBLE. A budget is nothing more than a health care manager's prediction of the future. The future being as

uncertain as it is, no budget can consistently be followed without periodic deviation from projected levels. The manager should refrain from overlooking opportunities to improve department operation because of a blind adherence to the budget.

3) DON'T EMPHASIZE SHORT-TERM RESULTS. In some instances, managers who are having difficulty meeting current budgetary guidelines may forgo the repair or purchase of vital equipment. Other managers may restrict subordinate working hours and subsequently increase them once the critical time period has passed. Taking temporary steps to solve long-term problems is seldom wise. Budgets should always be developed with a forecast of future events and allow the manager to adapt to change.

4) BUDGETS CAN BE MOTIVATIONAL. Budgets establish standards of performance. A properly designed method of budgeting can be motivational if the manager is rewarded for falling within acceptable parameters. Budgets which are considered motivational establish levels of managerial performance that are reasonably high but obtainable.

Most health care organizations will follow the traditional method of incremental budgeting, the zero base budget, or some similar method which is better tailored to their needs. The primary benefit of budgeting is that it allows goals to be expressed in financial terms so performance can more easily be evaluated. Deviations from established standards are readily measurable and provide a basis for corrective action. Those managers who develop and utilize good budgeting skills are valuable assets to the health care organization.

FINANCIAL ANALYSIS OF AN ORGANIZATION

Understanding the internal operations of a health care organization is vital to developing a successful career in health care management. Knowing some of the underlying reasons why top managers do the things they do comes from understanding the financial aspects of the organization. Financial statements present an analysis of the uses of organizational resources, the flow of goods, money, and services to, within, and from the organization.[5] Financial statement preparation is generally performed on an annual basis. The purpose of financial statement preparation is to indicate the financial events that have transpired since the preparation of the last set of financial statements.

Analyzing the financial performance of an organization can be a very difficult process which, to be done properly, would extend far beyond the scope of this book. A brief summary of the two most frequently encountered financial statements is provided. The balance sheet and income statement are two methods of financial analysis which allow the manager to determine whether the organization is growing or changing and, if so, how fast and in what directions.

The Balance Sheet

The balance sheet is a financial statement that reports the financial position of the health care organization at a specific point in time. The balance sheet is generally dated on the close of the last business day, such as December thirty-first. The last day of December is usually chosen because it reflects the end of the business year for most organizations. Figure 11-1 provides an example of the balance sheet format.

The balance sheet is divided into two parts: those resources owned by the health care organization called assets, and those owed to others called liabilities. The residual interest in the health care organization is called owner's equity. Owner's equity is determined by subtracting the organization's liabilities from its assets. If the health care organization is profitable, owner's equity will increase. Conversely, if the organization loses money, owner's equity will decline. The most important point to recognize is that what the organization owns is recognized as an asset. Liabilities are what the organization owes to others.

Income Statement

The income statement is a financial statement that demonstrates the financial changes that have occurred in the health care organization as a result of its operations over time. The income statement cannot be considered the same as a balance sheet. The income statement demonstrates changes that have taken place over a specific period of time, usually one year. The balance sheet, on the other hand, reflects the organization's financial position at a point in time.

The income statement will report the relative success or failure of the health care organization during the period under examination. It will

SMITHTOWN HOSPITAL

Balance Sheet – December 31, 19XX

ASSETS			LIABILITIES		
Current Assets			**Current Liabilities**		
Cash	500,000		Accounts Payable	600,000	
Accounts Receivable	100,000		Taxes Payable	400,000	
Inventory	10,000		Loan Payable	3,000,000	
Prepaid Expenses	5,000				
Total Current Assets		$ 615,000	Total Current Liabilities		$ 4,000,000
Fixed Assets			**Long Term Liabilities**		
Land		500,000	Bank Loan	1,000,000	
Building	5,000,000				
Less Accumulated Depreciation	1,000,000		Total Liabilities		$ 5,000,000
		4,000,000			
Equipment	500,000		Owner's Equity		$ 515,000
Less Accumulated Depreciation	100,000				
		400,000			
Total Fixed Assets		$ 4,900,000			
TOTAL ASSETS		$ 5,515,000	**TOTAL LIABILITIES + OWNER'S EQUITY**		$ 5,515,000

Figure 11-1.

identify whether revenues were greater or less than expenses. Most health care organizations prepare income statements annually, but it is not uncommon for organizations to develop monthly, quarterly, or semi-annual statements. Figure 11-2 is an example of a simplified income statement.

When examining the income statement for a business organization or similar activity, it will become apparent that the statement can be divided into three categories. The categories are: revenues, expenses, and net income. Revenues are recognized as the total services provided by the health care organization. A total hip replacement performed today, for example, is recognized as revenue even though the patient may not pay for the services rendered for several weeks. From the moment the hospital treats a patient it can claim an increase in revenue.

Financial Report for the Year Ending December 31, 19xx

Sources of funds:

Patient services		$ 120,722,369
Charitable or uncompensated services	$ 9,314,669	
Less than full payment from Medicare, Medicade and other government programs	22,616,804	31,931,473
		$ 88,790,896

Additional funds:

Contributions, investment income and gain or loss on disposal of assets		1,044,280
Nonpatient sources including cafeteria sales, purchase discounts and employee sales		1,240,697
		$ 91,075,873

Application of funds:

Wages and salaries		$ 34,006,914
Supplies and other services		35,044,120
Interest		4,036,478
Depreciation		7,316,387
Florida indigent tax		1,358,436
		$ 81,762,335

Excess of revenues over expenses:

To use for working capital, new equipment and improvements in salaries and benefits		$ 9,313,538

Figure 11-2.

Expenses are the costs the health care organization incurs while offering its services. In the total hip replacement example, the expenses associated with the operation would include the cost for sterilizing the surgical instruments, nursing salaries, time allotted for the procedure itself, as well as all other related costs. Expenses are also recorded at the time they are incurred.

Net income is the excess of revenue over expenses. When revenues exceed the expenses incurred, the organization has a net profit. If, however, the opposite is true (expenses exceed revenues), the organization incurs a loss. At the end of the accounting period, all organizational expenses are subtracted from revenues to determine whether the organization has made an overall profit or has suffered a loss.

BREAK-EVEN ANALYSIS

Suppose you are interested in approaching your supervisor and requesting the purchase of a new rehabilitative machine for your department. You know the equipment is worthwhile, will be highly in demand, and will easily pay for itself. As you approach the supervisor you develop a sense of insecurity because you have no hard data to prove the equipment will be financially worthwhile. How do you demonstrate that the revenues generated from the use of the equipment will more than cover the cost? There are a number of ways to substantiate the value of the equipment to the organization. One of the most simple is that of the break-even analysis formula.

The break-even formula is an analytical technique for examining the various relationships between fixed costs, variable costs, and the revenues generated by the organization. The basic assumption behind break-even analysis is that management would ideally like to make a profit on its services, but, if that is not possible, they would at least like to minimize their losses. The break-even formula allows managers to ascertain the amount of profit or loss that will occur based upon a projected level of patient care.

The break-even point is that point where the revenue generated in providing patient care services is equal to the cost of providing those services. In computing the break-even point there are several terms which must be identified.

P = Profit	Profit is the amount of income the organization generates above expenses.
R = Total Revenue	Total revenue is the dollar amount generated from the services provided.
C = Total Cost	Total cost is a monetary figure which represents the sum of fixed and variable costs.
F = Fixed Cost	An expense that will remain unchanged, at least in the short run, regardless of the quantity of services provided.
X = Units/Services	The letter "X" represents the number of services or units of a service provided.
S = Price	Price is the dollar amount charged by the organization for the service or unit of a service provided.
V = Variable Cost	Variable cost is the monetary figure representing the costs to the organization each time the service or unit of service is provided. When few services are provided, these costs are low. When the number of services provided increase, these costs will also rise.

To compute the break-even point, the terms must first be transformed into a mathematical statement. For example profit is determined by subtracting the total cost from total revenue.

$$P = \text{Total Revenue} - \text{Total Cost}$$
$$P = R - C$$

Total revenue is determined by multiplying the number of units of service provided by the organization's charge for that service.

$$\text{Total Revenue} = \text{Price} \times \text{Units/Service}$$
$$R = SX$$

Total cost is the sum of fixed and variable costs. The variable cost is determined by multiplying the number of services provided by the costs to the organization for providing those services.

$$\text{Total Cost} = \text{Fixed Cost} + (\text{Cost Per Service} \times \text{Number of Services})$$
$$C = F + VX$$

The relationships between profit, total revenue, and total costs are combined as follows:

$$P = R - C$$
$$P = SX - (F + VX)$$

This equation is the break-even formula. It conveniently expresses the relationships that exist between volume, fixed cost, variable cost, and the charge per unit of service. Its use is illustrated in the following health care example.

A physical therapy supervisor desires to purchase a new $15,000 whirlpool for the department. The supervisor estimates fixed costs including insurance, property taxes and salaries could be applied to the unit at $1,500 annually. Each of these fixed costs are expected to remain constant throughout the next year. The sum of the fixed costs is $16,500. Each time the 200-gallon whirlpool is filled it will cost approximately eight cents per gallon for a total of $16 per visit. The supervisor plans to charge $25 per treatment. With this information, the mathematical model can be used to answer several questions: What will be the profit if 500 patients are treated?

$$P = SX - (F + VX)$$
$$P = 25(500) - [16,500 + 16(500)]$$
$$P = 12,500 - [16,500 + 8,000] = -\$12,000$$

With a projected $12,000 loss, how many patients must the department treat in order to break even? To break even implies the profit equals zero. To solve for "X" (the number of patients treated), "P" must equal zero.

$$P = SX - (F + VX)$$
$$O = 25X - (16,500 + 16X)$$
$$O = 9X - 16,500$$
$$X = 1834 \text{ Patient Treatments}$$

Figure 11-3 demonstrates the graphic solution to the problem. The use of break-even analysis requires algebra and common sense to solve simple managerial problems. In this case, the more patients referred to physical therapy, the sooner the equipment will begin to evidence a profitable return on investment.

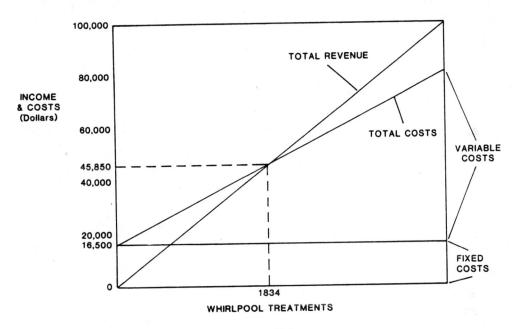

Figure 11-3.

BUDGETING IN PERSPECTIVE

Budgets and break-even points are invaluable to the supervisor in controlling costs and in estimating the revenues generated in a department. The supervisor has the responsibility for ensuring the department makes a profit and reaches its objectives and goals. Nevertheless, the manager must remain alert to some of the variables which can be affected by the budget.

It is not uncommon for subordinates to develop defensive attitudes towards the budgeting process. Many times management blames the budget for an inability to give raises. In other instances budgets become real or hypothetical barriers for the purchase of new equipment. Health care managers can lower their credibility by continually blaming the budget for their inability to get things accomplished. If subordinates know the department is making a profit, they will find it very difficult to go for prolonged periods without being rewarded. A subordinate is unlikely to find satisfaction in an organization where salaries are low and profits are high. As such, the budgetary system should be looked upon as a method for providing timely and accurate feedback. Each employee should be advised about the quality of their work and recognized for the contribution they make to the organization.

REFERENCES

1. William O. Cleverley, Essentials of Health Care Finance (Rockville, MD: Aspen Publication, 1986), pp. 254–255.
2. A. Shick, "A Death in the Bureaucracy: The Demise of Federal PPB," Public Administration Review, 26 (March–April 1973), pp. 146–156.
3. "What It Means to Build a Budget from Zero," Business Week, April 18, 1977, pp. 160–164, "What Zero-Base Budgeting is and How Carter Wants to Use It," U.S. News & World Report, April 25, 1977, pp. 91–93, P. Phyrr,"Zero-Base Budgeting," Harvard Business Review, 48, (November--December 1970), pp. 111–121, L. Cheek, Zero Base Budgeting Comes of Age (New York: American Management Association, 1977).
4. "What It Means to Build a Budget from Zero."
5. W. F. Frese & R. K. Mautz, "Financial Reporting—By Whom?" Harvard Business Review (March–April 1972), pp. 6–12.

Chapter Twelve

THE MANAGERIAL DECISION-MAKING PROCESS

Decision making is an integral part of the job of every physical therapist. Each day decisions must be made concerning the welfare of patients and the rehabilitative avenues which are to be pursued. Decision making is also an important aspect of the job of a health care manager. Being placed in a managerial position is, without a doubt, based on your specialized ability to make sound decisions. The quality of decisions that managers reach is the yardstick of their effectiveness.[1]

The process of making a decision is not a fixed technique. The decision-making process is dynamic and ongoing, partially because of the varying backgrounds, educational experiences, and life-styles which each of us come from. No matter how seemingly insignificant a decision may appear, it will be somewhat different from the one before it.

The focus of this chapter is on the managerial decision-making process. Managerial decisions all have a certain number of elements in common. Each decision is made against a background of information and involves a certain number of key elements. This chapter describes and analyzes decision making in terms that reflect the way people decide a course of action based upon the information they have received. The information may be received from the organization itself or from the behavior of groups or individuals within and outside the health care organization.

LEVELS OF MANAGERIAL DECISION MAKING

Managers at all levels in the health care organization are responsible for making decisions. Depending on the manager's position in the organization's hierarchy, the type of decisions made, and their eventual impact on the organization will vary. Decisions made improperly at key levels in the organization can be costly. Understanding who is responsible for decision making is therefore an important managerial requirement.

Those health care managers who occupy positions in lower levels of management normally make more decisions during a given period of time than do health care managers at higher levels. Many of the decisions made at lower levels are considered programmed. That is, they deal directly with the daily operations of providing patient care and department operation. Many of these decisions are based upon established policies, procedures, and methods of operation. The decisions follow what has previously been determined to be the best course of action.

Middle level managers in a health care organization make even fewer decisions than those at the primary levels of supervision. Here, the manager is concerned with allocating resources or deciding how many personnel each department may have. One of the primary decision-making responsibilities of middle level managers is to decide how to implement the objectives and goals which were developed as part of top management's decision making.

Top managers make still fewer decisions than middle level managers. Their decisions do, however, have a more long-term and significant impact on the health care organization. The decisions top manager's make will affect all levels of the organization (see Figure 12-1). A decision made by the executives of the W. T. Grant Company led to the eventual demise of the organization.

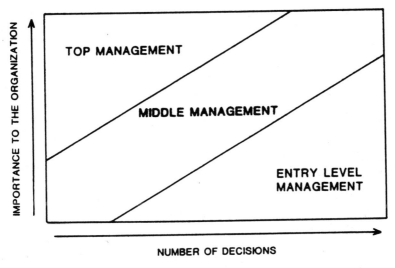

Figure 12-1.

In 1972, W. T. Grant was the country's seventeenth largest retailer, with 1200 stores and $38 million dollars in profits. The top management at W. T. Grant decided the best growth strategy would be a rapid increase in the number of stores. Between the years of 1969 and 1973, W. T. Grant opened another 369 stores. In 1974, the company lost $177 million. The huge loss and the company's eventual bankruptcy were attributed to that top management decision.[2]

TYPES OF DECISIONS

Each of us has been placed in situations where decision making was not considered a complex task. In other instances, making the proper decision was not well defined and straightforward. One of the most critical aspects of making a proper decision is determining what type of decision will be required. Herbert Simion distinguishes between two types of decisions: those which are programmed and those which are considered non-programmed.[3]

1) PROGRAMMED DECISIONS. Those decisions which are considered programmable are fairly repetitive and routine. In most situations, definite and systematic procedures have been established for making the proper choice. A large majority of the decisions made by members of management in a health care organization are programmable. That is, they are based on established policies, procedures, rules and methods of organization. For example, most hospitals have developed standardized methods for computing payrolls, admitting patients, scheduling surgery, or for hiring new employees. Here, the health care manager's job is simply to judge whether a decision is programmed and ensure the decision and the various programs are properly implemented.

2) NON-PROGRAMMED DECISIONS. Those decisions which are non-programmed are often unique and have no established procedure for handling a problem. The problem may be new or has not arisen in exactly the same manner before. The decision which has to be made must be done with fewer rules, procedures, or guidelines to follow. Decisions such as these require considerably more judgment on the part of the manager.

Although the two classifications of decision making are broad, they do have important implications for managers. The director of physical therapy must recognize routine decisions and take appropriate action without utilizing unnecessary resources. The health care manager should not waste valuable working hours or resources on routine decision making. On the other hand, the manager must identify those decisions which are unique and will require additional organizational resources. Figure 12-2 provides an example of some of the decisions made by the physical therapy supervisor.

Most health care managers, especially those in entry level or middle management, make decisions based on specific rules or guidelines for handling a problem. Top management makes a majority of the non-programmed decisions. The nature of the problem, its frequency, and the degree of certainty surrounding the problem will often dictate the level of management assigned to make the decision.

TYPES OF DECISIONS

	PROGRAMED DECISIONS	NON PROGRAMED DECISIONS
PROBLEM	Routine, frequently encountered and repetitive	Considerable uncertainty rarely, if ever encountered
PROCEDURE	Refer to organizations policies, procedures and rules	Requires creative problem solving
EXAMPLES	Procedure for scheduling patients Rules concerning employee smoking	Request for obtaining highly controversial rehabilitation equipment Construction of a new department

Figure 12-2.

MANAGERIAL DECISION MAKING UNDER CONDITIONS OF CERTAINTY, RISK, AND UNCERTAINTY

Managers make decisions in health care organizations as part of the process of reaching desired objectives and goals. Some of the decisions made have profound effects upon the health care services offered and the way the organization operates. Reaching a decision requires a prediction of the future based upon the availability of adequate information. The information which is available, and its accuracy, determines whether decisions are made under conditions of certainty, risk, or uncertainty. Figure 12-3 demonstrates how available information affects the riskiness of a decision.

Conditions of Certainty

When a manager possesses enough information in order to predict the future, a decision can be made under conditions of certainty. When the decision is eventually made, it is very likely the desired outcome will be achieved. Some decisions made under conditions of certainty are quite simple and require little thought, whereas others are more complex and

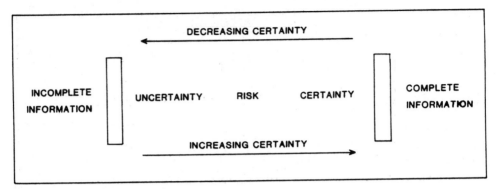

Figure 12-3.

must be examined in depth. If, for example, the manager decides to have a staff meeting at 9:00 A.M. tomorrow, the chances are quite good that all the staff will be present. It is important to recognize that even under conditions of certainty the future, as projected, may be subject to change. A subordinate may become ill and not attend the manager's scheduled meeting.

Conditions of Risk

When conditions of risk are present, the manager has at least a partial estimate of the potential outcomes for each available alternative. Managerial decision making under conditions of risk is probably the most common of all.[4] The element of risk can be defined as the probability of a desired outcome. Probability is a statistical term which identifies the chance or percentage of times an outcome or result would occur if allowed to happen. In health care, malpractice insurance premiums are established based upon the degree of risk or likelihood of a lawsuit. The profession of physical therapy has very low malpractice insurance premiums as compared to medical doctors who specialize in neurosurgery or orthopaedic medicine. Those health care professionals who practice in high-risk specialities are often assigned high liability premiums.

Conditions of Uncertainty

When conditions are uncertain, the decision maker has no knowledge of the likelihood of an outcome. If the manager is presented with a large number of factors to consider and each of these factors is in a constant state of flux, the manager will have a more difficult time arriving at a decision. When presented with this situation, the manager may have to rely on his or her judgment, experience, and intuition to select the best alternative. For example, the owner of a private practice may have perceived the need to establish a back school in his or her community. In trying to arrive at an implementation decision, the practitioner carefully evaluated the local community and the potential medical referral sources. Having been unable to obtain any firm commitments regarding its usage, the manager must make a decision based solely on judgment and intuition. All attempts to obtain concrete information have failed and the practitioner must now personally assess how valuable the back school could be.

THE LIMITS TO DECISION MAKING

When the manager is searching for the solution to a problem, it is sometimes possible to find the solution without first identifying all the possible alternatives. This approach to decision making is called *satisficing.* The manager may cease working on a problem as soon as a satisfactory solution is found. The outcome of managerial decisions of this type is a satisfactory decision rather than an optimal decision.

March and Simion have observed that rarely are decision makers concerned with making optimal decisions; consequently, satisficing is what generally occurs.[5] They remark that optimizing is like searching in a haystack for the sharpest needle, but satisficing is like searching a haystack for a needle that is sharp enough to sew with. This has particular applications to the health care manager, especially when searching for additional staff. With the relative shortage of physical therapists a manager might, for example, hire the first applicant for a position who has the necessary qualifications rather than continuing to search for the best employee.

The concept of bounded rationality occurs when the available alternatives are so numerous that management cannot possibly evaluate them all. The problem may be so complex and solutions so numerous that even by using the most sophisticated computer, the manager cannot possibly consider all solutions. When problems are so complex or have an endless number of extraneous variables, a manager may choose to reduce the complexity of the problem to a level where the possible alternatives can be handled.

For the health care manager it is important to clearly distinguish between the concepts of satisficing and bounded rationality. Satisficing is a deliberate choice to limit the number of alternatives to be evaluated before the selection of a solution. Bounded rationality is a limit naturally imposed because of the complex nature of the situation. With bounded rationality there is a natural limit on human ability to handle complex situations. Limits arise due to an individual's inability to process large amounts of information.

Bounded discretion is a limitation which has been placed on optimal decision making by either moral or ethical constraints.[6] Following the concept of bounded discretion, a decision maker will limit the possible number of actions to those which fall within the bounds of acceptable moral and ethical standards. For example, some possible alternatives for a surgeon faced with a malpractice suit might include: fighting the suit, giving in to the patient's allegations, altering the patient's chart, destroying the chart, or attempting to sway the opinions of others who may have witnessed the alleged error. Although some of the solutions may seem extreme, they could outwardly appear quite logical to the physician, depending on his or her bounded discretion.

STEPS IN THE DECISION-MAKING PROCESS

For decisions which are unprogrammable and involve a significant element of risk, the health care manager may experience considerable stress when attempting to reach an optimal decision. The stress associated with decision making under conditions of risk or uncertainty can be reduced by following a simple six-step process. The steps are shown in Figure 12-4.

Thoroughly Diagnose the Situation

The key element to solving any problem is understanding what the problem is. The physical therapist must be especially careful to fully diagnose what is happening. It is easy to select one prominent symptom and label it as the cause of the problem. Medical doctors, as office employers, often have high turnovers of personnel. When asked why, many doctors respond, "In health care the turnover of personnel has always been high. Nothing can be done to change that." When fully investigated, however, many doctors are surprised to discover the prob-

---

STEPS IN THE DECISION MAKING PROCESS

---

1. Thoroughly Diagnose the Situation

2. Develop Alternative Solutions

3. Evaluate the Alternatives

4. Select the Alternative

5. Implement the Solution

6. Evaluation and Control

Figure 12-4.

lem with turnover may be representative of an underlying cause rather than a symptom and characteristic of the industry.

The process of problem identification can begin by locating deviations from established objectives and then looking for the reasons behind them.[7] The health care manager must carefully examine historical data which shows changes in current behavior as compared to past performance. By reviewing historical data and established plans the manager can obtain information which clearly demonstrates that objectives and goals have not been achieved.

One of the difficulties in clearly diagnosing the situation has to do with the manager's possible reluctance to recognize a problem exists. Individual perception may cloud or selectively distort the true meaning in a situation. Perception is the process the person uses to select, organize, translate, and interpret stimuli to influence behavior and form attitudes. Perception involves acquiring knowledge about specific events or objects and interpreting this knowledge in the light of previous experience.

Perception is important to the health care manager, since employees often have different views of what performance is expected. Their views may not be in agreement with those of the supervisor. The manager must recognize this potential problem and respect differing views of a situation. Only then can the manager develop alternative solutions which recognize all aspects of a problem.

Develop Alternative Solutions

Once a problem has been clearly identified, the next step is to identify the alternative solutions. Developing alternative solutions can be done by either following the traditional method or by use of a more creative approach. Following the traditional method recognizes the use of logic. Here, the manager examines the problem and develops alternatives with the idea in mind of simply solving the problem. The problem with logical alternative solution development is that the organization may be overlooking the opportunity to be creative and stimulate fresh ideas within the organization.

Creativity can be important to health care managers. Organizations can help foster creativity in management by:[8]

1) BUFFERING. Creative decisions are more risky than those developed by traditional methods. The health care manager can look for ways to implement creative ideas without threatening the security of the health care organization.

2) ORGANIZATIONAL TIME-OUTS. If the problem requires a significant amount of time and effort to solve, the manager may request time away from normal duties. This provides the manager with an opportunity to think things through without continual interruption.

3) INTUITION. No idea should be haphazardly rejected. Even when it is obvious that an idea will not work, give its creator a chance to discover it for him or herself.

4) INNOVATIVE ATTITUDES. Encourage all organizational members, from the highest to lowest levels, to participate in developing possible solutions.

5) INNOVATIVE ORGANIZATIONAL STRUCTURES. Encourage subordinates to interact with members of other departments. Recommend they work as a team on solving patient- and non-patient-related problems.

Evaluate the Alternatives

Each alternative must be considered for its sense of realism and feasibility. Evaluating the realism of an alternative includes deciding whether or not the alternative can be effectively implemented in the health care organization. The implementation of some alternatives may take more effort than the organization can commit. Feasibility includes evaluating whether the organization has the time or necessary resources to implement the alternatives. An organization must consider whether the potential profit contribution will make the alternative worth adopting. The evaluation of alternative solutions can be conducted using the following guidelines:

1) DOUBLE CHECK THE INFORMATION WHICH HAS BEEN PROVIDED. If the search for an alternative is limited by time, there is a tendency for the decision to be based not on valid data but on opinions. A supervisor who is under time constraints may accept a subordinate's evaluation of a problem without questioning the information provided. It is not that subordinates are pushing for the implementation of their alternative as much as it is a willingness to be of assistance to the supervisor. Even when the data provided appears to be sound, it must be verified.

2) ENCOURAGE SPONTANEITY IN ALTERNATIVE DEVELOPMENT. Some of the best alternatives are those which required little or no thought to develop. Managers often resist "novel" ideas because they feel they will have a difficult time explaining them to supervisors.

3) UNDERSTAND THE CONSEQUENCES OF EACH ALTERNATIVE. Especially when under time pressures for a solution, a manager may look at an alternative through "rose-colored glasses." Every decision presents a certain element of risk. The more riskier the decision, the more likely unintended consequences will result if things do not turn out as planned. Always consider both the good and bad points of any alternative and plan what to do should events transpire other than as planned.

Select the Alternative

Once all of the alternatives have been evaluated, the next step will involve selecting a course of action. The alternative chosen will be based upon the information that is available at the time the decision must be made. Considering most managers are influenced to at least some degree by satisficing and bounded rationality, reaching the optimal decision may be difficult. In selecting an alternative solution the health care manager should consider the following:

1) DO NOT RUSH ALTERNATIVE SELECTION. Although a great number of excellent decisions are made with little or no thought, rapid decision making does increase the chances of error. Following a

thorough and logical thought process helps reduce the chances of error in managerial decision making.

2) BE FLEXIBLE IN DECISION MAKING. The health care manager should avoid becoming a creature of habit in decision making. To do so requires a commitment to remain open to new ideas and creative solutions. Never entertain the idea that you are the only one capable or qualified to make the decision. In many cases it will be the subordinate who will be charged with implementing the managerial directive. Therefore, the manager must encourage subordinate involvement.

3) ALTERNATIVES DO NOT HAVE TO BE INTELLECTUAL. One of the key elements to success in health care management is the use of common sense. Management in health care is considerably more an art than a science. As such, the selection of an alternative may require the use of creativity and imagination rather than a reliance on hard-core data.

Implement the Solution

Those health care professionals who are successful in health care management are confident of the decisions they make and anxious to see them implemented. The announcement of a managerial decision should not be done in a halfhearted or apologetic manner. A manager who is indecisive creates uncertainty in the minds of others. Many good decisions are rendered ineffective by improper implementation at the management level.

Evaluation and Control

The implementation of a decision requires substantially more than just giving the appropriate orders. Effective implementation of a decision must include the periodic measurement of the expected results. The manager should not fail to express continued interest in the problem once a solution has been implemented. Employees will be quick to recognize a manager who gives orders but never examines the results.

Control, as discussed in Chapter One, is the process of comparing actual performance against predetermined objectives and goals. When performance does not meet with established objectives and goals, corrective action must be taken. The process of managerial control consists of four steps. As is shown in Figure 12-5, managerial control can be an important guiding principle to all health care managers. Each is discussed in the following:

1) ESTABLISHING PERFORMANCE CRITERIA. All managerial decision making should include establishing standards or reference points to which actual performance can be compared. When decisions are implemented, the results of the implementation should be easily ascertainable.

2) MEASURE INDIVIDUAL PERFORMANCE. Ascertaining performance may be through the use of qualitative or quantitative measures or some combination of the two. Performance may also be assessed by using either short- or long-term measurements. Some of the more common ways of measuring performance include the following criteria:

Effectiveness	Satisfaction
Attendance	Motivation
Retention	Innovation
Productivity	Adaptability
Efficiency	Development
Profit	Quality
Growth	Safety

STEPS IN THE CONTROL PROCESS

Establish Performance criteria

Measure individual performance

Compare performance to established standards

Take corrective action

Figure 12-5.

Of the criteria listed above, it is important to recognize the differences between two very important items: that of efficiency and effectiveness. These terms have received considerable attention in management literature because of the increasing demands organizations have placed on their managers to achieve objectives and goals. In other words, there is a strong and growing emphasis on managerial performance.

Peter Drucker has stated that efficiency means "doing things right" and effectiveness means "doing the right things."[9] Efficiency is an engineering concept that concerns the relationship between "inputs" and "outputs." For example, the efficiency of a physical therapy treatment session for a patient with adhesive capsulities can be measured by evaluating the increase in range of motion achieved in comparison with the expenditure of effort by the physical therapist. The input would be the therapist's time and effort, while the output would be the increase in range of motion.

From the standpoint of management, efficiency may concern a manager's level of output (the accomplishment of departmental objectives and goals) with a given level of input. A health care manager who can minimize the cost of resources used to operate a department and achieve established objectives and goals would be functioning efficiently.

Effectiveness is how well the health care organization achieves its objectives and goals over time. To be effective the management of a health care organization must have the ability to adapt, to implement changes, reach objectives, and serve its mission. An organization is effective if it can respond to changes required in order to survive. Those managers who are considered effective select the correct approaches to problems and achieve their desired goals.

3) COMPARE PERFORMANCE TO ESTABLISHED STANDARDS. The standards established by the manager are the basis by which performance of the organization and its personnel are judged. When performance does not meet the predetermined objectives and goals, the manager must take corrective action.

4) TAKE CORRECTIVE ACTION. A manager who desires to take corrective action is interested in changing the performance of an organization and its members. Corrective action can be applied to improve financial performance, absenteeism, turnover, productivity, and safety. Control must be present at all levels throughout the organization.

FACTORS AFFECTING THE DECISION-MAKING PROCESS

Decisions are profoundly influenced by value judgments. No decision can be made without considering the impact an individual's values have upon the ultimate decision. A value is an individual's wants, desires, dislikes or preferences for a specific thing, condition, preferred outcome, or situation. A value also represents what the individual thinks is fair, right, or desirable. It can, therefore, be expressed as an opinion.

No managerial decision can be made without some influence being provided by the external environment, the organization, and the individual values of the health care manager. A manager cannot objectively look at what the organization wants to do without being partially influenced by what he or she would like to do.

Values not only affect the health care manager, they also influence the subordinate. In recent years, value differences among people, professions, and cultures have received increasing attention from behavioral scientists and practicing managers. One of the more useful approaches to managerial values is the one that classifies them into six value orientations.[10]

1) THEORETICAL. An individual with a strong theoretical value orientation is interested in the discovery of the truth and a systematic ordering of knowledge. Such people demonstrate interests in areas that are empirical and rational.
2) ECONOMIC. Those individuals who present an interest in economic values are oriented toward the practical aspects of work. They are interested in the efficient treatment of patients, the proper use of resources (equipment and manpower), and the creation of wealth.
3) AESTHETIC. A person with a strong interest in aesthetic values is concerned primarily with symmetry, grace, and harmony. They may recognize and express interest in the artistic features of an object or event.
4) SOCIAL VALUES. The dominant interests of a person with a high concern for social values is to value people as ends rather than as means. They tend to be kind, sympathetic, unselfish, value people and warm human relationships.
5) POLITICAL. A person who possesses dominant political values is oriented towards power and influence. The person may be quite competitive and adhere strongly to political values.
6) RELIGIOUS. Those individuals with high religious values have an orientation toward God, strong religious values, and work to build satisfying relations with the environment.

It is also well recognized that an individual's values are strongly influenced by his or her immediate culture. Those people who are influential in the individual's life will also have influence on their value development. Values, as such, are learned by the individual through interactions with parents, teachers, friends, and other health care professionals. The physical therapist's approach to patient care and behavior exercised while in a health care management position will be influenced by individual values.

Emotions may also play a vital role in the effectiveness of decision making. A decision based primarily on emotions is one in which the individual relied on subjective feelings rather than on substantiated facts. Decisions made based on emotion include those made when the individual is scared, happy, or angry. Obviously, decisions based on these emotions are subject to error, since they may have little or no hard data to reinforce the decision-making process.

Rational decisions are based on objective facts. A manager who strives to make a rational decision does so based on logic or on an analysis of the information which has been provided. Arriving at a totally rational decision is rather idealistic. A health care manager cannot know all of the possible alternatives, their potential consequences, and eliminate the influence of emotions. When striving to make a rational decision the manager must ask the following questions:

1) How much does each alternative contribute to reaching the primary objective or goal? Does the most rational of the available decisions conform with organizational policies and procedures, or will changes have to be made?
2) Will the rational decision be cost effective? Some decisions, although very logical and rational, are too costly when compared to the benefits derived.
3) How well can the decision be implemented? A rational decision will be ineffective if implemented in an irrational manner.

Figure 12-6 shows the relative differences between emotional and rational decision making. On the far right, decisions are based on objective facts and scientific evidence, thus resulting in less chance of managerial error. Those decisions on the far left are subject to a high degree of error.

MANAGERIAL DECISION MAKING WITH SUBORDINATES

A good portion of health care manager's time is spent working directly with other health care professionals. Therefore, much of the decision making a manager does should be influenced by those who will be most closely associated with the eventual outcome. Practicing health care

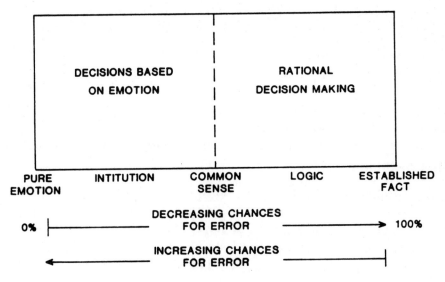

Figure 12-6.

managers are frequently in need of specific techniques that will act as guides when others are to be included in decision making. Three techniques have been found to be very useful in increasing the creative capability of a group in generating ideas, understanding problems, and reaching better decisions. The three techniques of particular value to health care managers are brainstorming, the Delphi technique, and the nominal group technique.

Brainstorming is a technique developed by Alex Osborne that has been available to managers for over forty years.[11] Brainstorming is a method designed to encourage the creative output of a group. The objective is to support the free flow of ideas while at the same time suspending all critical judgments. The basic rules of the Osborne technique are as follows:

1) NO IDEA SHOULD BE CRITICIZED. The purpose of the group is to generate ideas, not discourage them through criticism.
2) NO IDEA IS TOO EXTREME. Outlandish ideas are welcomed.
3) THE GREATER THE NUMBER OF IDEAS, THE BETTER. Members of the group are encouraged to offer as many ideas and potential solutions as possible.
4) BUILDING ON THE IDEAS OF OTHERS IS ALSO ENCOURAGED. If one member of the group develops a particularly good idea, others

are encouraged to add to it or expand upon it. Each idea developed belongs to the group, not solely to the individual.

The ideal length of time for a brainstorming session is not less than twenty minutes, nor more than one hour. No more than five to ten people should be involved in any one session. If, after the specified period of time, the solution has not been found, the brainstorming session may be resumed at additional idea-generating sessions. To properly use the brainstorming method the manager should implement the following guidelines:

1) At the beginning of each session, the manager should review the basic rules. New members of the group should be introduced and informed of the events that have transpired thus far. The ideas which have been developed should also be available for further discussion. The use of a chalkboard is excellent for listing new ideas.

2) If there are periods when the group becomes misdirected or loses sight of the issue, the manager should repeat the problem and ask once again for ideas. It is the manager's responsibility to combine ideas that are similar and encourage an in-depth thought process.

3) Each idea presented should be summarized by the health care manager. This helps to ensure the proposed solution is understood by all group members. During the discussion of ideas, the manager should feel free to interrupt any presenter who talks for too long. No one member of the group should dominate the discussion or push his or her ideas onto everyone else.

4) The health care manager should refrain from becoming an active participant in the brainstorming process. Although the manager still performs the primary function of guiding and directing the group, active participation may lead to reduced group productivity.

5) Above all, the manager must prevent an individual's ideas from being judged, criticized, or haphazardly disregarded. The manager serves to keep the group focused and help develop individual members. A member should not be "put down" for his or her ideas or proposed solutions.

The Delphi technique is a method for securing the consensus of a group of experts regarding their predictions of a future event or assessment of current needs.[12] The group of experts do not have physical contact with one another but instead interact through the use of questionnaires. The members are considered knowledgeable about the issue but work anonymously, in a step-by-step process, to solve problems. The Delphi technique works as follows:

1) The manager selects a group of people who he or she considers knowledgeable about a particular problem or issue. The panel may consist of people who are members of the organization and/or those who do not have direct ties to the organization. The panel members do not have to know one another.

2) The manager develops a questionnaire about the particular problem to be solved and mails one to each panel member. The panel member is asked to anonymously complete the questionnaire and return it to the manager. The manager then pools the various ideas and suggestions and prepares a feedback report.

3) The feedback summary along with a second questionnaire is then sent to each panel member.

4) Upon receipt, each panel member is requested to re-evaluate their earlier responses and the responses of other members. They are then requested to vote on the ideas and generate any new ideas which may lead to the optimal solution.

5) The process is continued until the manager feels enough information has been obtained in order to make a decision.

6) Once the decision has been made, the manager reports the findings back to group members.

One of the primary advantages of the Delphi technique is that there is no interaction among panel members. When a group of experts come together to consider a problem or issue, there is always the chance that one member may dominate the discussion and the decision-making process. This is especially true when experts contain a mix of educational backgrounds and/or experience concerning the issue. An individual who considers him or herself as an expert may spend more time defending a thought process or decision rather than working with others towards group consensus.

As can be imagined, the primary disadvantage to the Delphi technique is that it is very time consuming. Obtaining rapid responses will vary depending on the person's interest in the subject matter and how much time they personally have to devote to the problem. It can also be quite time consuming to analyze all of the information received and reach a consensus. Obviously, the Delphi technique would not be appropriate for rapid decision making.

The nominal group technique is a structured group meeting designed to stimulate creative decision making. The technique has gained increasing recognition in the health, social service and educational sectors of this country.[13] Nominal group technique is designed to stimulate creative decision making where members of the group lack agreement on a problem or do not have sufficient knowledge to solve it. The idea is to have them pool thought processes and discover a satisfactory course of action. A meeting following the nominal group technique would be conducted as follows:[14]

1) Each member of the group silently expresses his or her ideas or solutions to a problem in writing. The members of the group may work together in the same room or be isolated in rooms away from one another.

2) After a short period of time (five to fifteen minutes), each member takes a few moments and shares his or her ideas with the other members. It is not uncommon for individual members of a group to have several ideas concerning a problem. If this occurs, ideas should be presented in a round-robin fashion with only one idea being presented at a time.

3) While each member of the group is sharing his or her ideas, one person, designated as the group recorder, should write the ideas on a chalkboard or flipchart in full view of the others. Ideas should not be matched with originators.

4) The group then discusses each idea. Throughout the discussion, the group should be encouraged to indicate support or non-support for each idea.

5) In the final phase, each member privately rank-orders their choices on a piece of paper. The decision is then mathematically determined.

The nominal group technique offers a number of advantages to the health care organization. When group members devote time toward writing out their ideas, there is likely to be a greater understanding of the problem and its possible ramifications. Members of the group do not simply solve the problem in their minds; they must put it in writing and be prepared to discuss their solutions with others. The nominal group technique also provides an opportunity for all group members to express ideas and thus contribute to the health care organization.

DECISION MAKING: LEFT BRAIN, RIGHT BRAIN

Physical therapists are well aware of the differences the two sides of the brain play in the function and rehabilitation of the human being. When one side of the brain has been traumatized, such as by a vascular lesion, it will often present one set of symptoms versus when the opposite side of the brain has been traumatized.[15] In the same fashion, a health care manager can also be influenced by which side of the brain is more dominant. For example, those individuals whose left brain is dominant are more analytical, systematic, sequential, and verbal. Individuals who are more right brain dominant will be more intuitive, visual, spatial, sensuous, and holistic.[16]

The complexities of the brain and the dominant features of each side have important implications for the health care manager.[17] Those individuals who are primarily left brain in orientation would be better suited for jobs which are analytical. Right brain people need to be in positions where they can exercise their ability to be conceptual and intuitive. In theory, right brain people should be more effective task leaders, since they pay more attention to the work group and its interactions. It has also been speculated that right brain people should be involved in creative activities such as formulating strategic objectives and goals, although little or no research has been conducted to support that idea.

DECISION MAKING AND MISTAKES

Health care managers make decisions affecting both patient and non-patient activities in an organization. Some of the decisions a manager makes will influence well beyond the boundries of the organization to include various segments of the surrounding community. Good managerial decision making can be considered both an art and a skill. Anyone who aspires to be successful in health care management must practice good decision-making skills.

Regardless of how hard the manager works at not making errors in judgment it is impossible to make the right decision everytime. There will be times when the manager regrettably makes the wrong decision. It is important for the manager to realize, however, that it is not the improper decision which has the greatest effect on the organization as much as it is the manager's handling the situation once the error has been made. Surprisingly, making errors in managerial decision making can be used to enhance the individuals credibility by following a few simple guidelines:

1) Do not hesitate to openly recognize you made an error. You should not, however, be overly conversive in apologizing for a mistake. Explain what went wrong as briefly as possible and allow others to fill in the details.

2) When it is clear an error has been made, move as swiftly as possible to warn all involved parties. Do not allow unintended consequences to occur.

3) Correct your mistakes. You should re-diagnose the problem and proceed, once again, through the proper decision-making steps.

4) Learn from your mistakes. The best way to improve your ability to make quality decisions is analyze why your own thought processes occurred as they did.

Finally, it is important for the health care manager to recognize that experience in making decisions will not always guarantee that future decisions will be any better or easier. The decisions you do make will, however, have a profound influence on those around you. Employees develop many of their own decision-making skills through careful observation of the health care manager. The better the decision-making skill of the supervisor, the more it will encourage subordinates. Guiding the subordinate through the decision-making process can pay substantial dividends. Once trained in proper decision-making techniques, employees will rely less on the supervisor in order to make proper decisions. This in turn will provide the manager with more time to devote to the other managerial functions.

REFERENCES

1. Bernard M. Bass, Organizational Decision Making (Homewood, IL: Richard D. Irwin, 1983).
2. "Investigating the Collapse of W. T. Grant," Business Week, July 19, 1976, pp. 60–62.
3. Herbert A. Simon, The New Science of Management Decision (New York: Harper & Row, 1960), pp. 5–6.
4. J. E. Hodder and H. E. Riggs, "Pitfalls in Evaluating Risky Projects," Harvard Business Review, January–February 1985, pp. 128–135.
5. J. G. March & H. A. Simon, Organizations (New York: Wiley, 1958).

6. F. A. Shull, A. L. Delbecq, & L.L. Cummings, Organizational Decision Making (New York: McGraw-Hill, 1970).

7. W. Pounds, "The Process of Problem Finding," Industrial Management Review, Fall 1969, pp. 1–19.

8. S. S. Gryskiewicz, "Restructing for Innovation," Issues and Observations, November 1981, p. 3.

9. P. F. Drucker, Managing for Results (New York: Harper & Row, 1964), p. 5.

10. G. Allport, P. Vernon, & G. Lindzey, Study of Values (Boston: Houghton Mifflin, 1960).

11. A. F. Osborne, Applied Imagination: Principles and Procedures for Creative Thinking (New York: Scribner's, 1941).

12. A. Delbecq, A. Van de Ven, and A. Gustason, Group Techniques for Program Planning: A Guide to Nominal Group, and Delphi Processes (Glenview, IL: Scott, Foresman, 1975).

13. Ibid.

14. Ibid.

15. Signe Brunnstrom, Movement Therapy in Hemiplegia (New York: Harper & Row, 1970).

16. R. E. Ornstein, The Psychology of Consciousness (New York: Viking Press, 1972), and S. P. Springer, Left Brain, Right Brain (San Francisco: W. H. Freeman, 1981).

17. This discussion is based on H. Mintzberg, "Planning on the Left and Managing on the Right," Harvard Business Review, July–August 1976, pp. 49–58., P. S. Nugent, "Management and Modes of Thought," Organizational Dynamics, Spring 1981, pp. 45–59.

Chapter Thirteen

MANAGERIAL CAREER DEVELOPMENT

M any physical therapists who read this book will be in managerial positions by the year 2000. The process of becoming a skilled health care manager requires early preparation. Whereas a career used to mean little more than a biweekly paycheck, today the health care professional recognizes it as much more. To be an effective health care manager, the physical therapist will undoubtedly require additional college course work that enhances not only technical skills but also decision-making, leadership, and human resources management skill.

Forecasting the management skills for the future is a difficult task. Alvin Toffler, author of *The Third Wave*, foresees a world in which managerial performance will be evaluated against a number of criteria that differ from the traditional concepts of profitability and profits. He predicts areas which will be measured include social, environmental, informational, political, and ethical indicators. There will be a movement away from the notion that "bigger is better" toward the idea of "appropriate scale."[1]

The general trend suggests that the physical therapist, as a supervisor, will need a careful blend of managerial and professional skills in order to be successful. Traditionally, the idea of mixing professional and management skills in the health care environment was viewed with skepticism. The belief was that management cannot be mixed with patient care. As the technological sophistication of medicine has increased, so has the demand for health care professionals with clinical competence and the ability to effectively lead organizations of all types.

The environment of today's health care organization is likely to change in the future. Changing events may cause specific managerial skills to take on different levels of importance over time. Even with the projected changes, a health care manager will still need basic competences in the technical, behavioral, and conceptual areas of management. A career in health care management includes those changes a person must make over time to adapt to economic, social and organizational conditions. This chapter focuses on how the physical therapist can take an active role in managing a career. Developing a career plays an important role in the way we view ourselves and the profession. Our sense of self-worth, identity, achievement, and eventual satisfaction are all affected by the career decisions we make.

MAKING EACH JOB A CHALLENGE

Success in health care management is directly related to your ability to select good administrative assignments. Early job experiences seem to be at least partially responsible for subsequent career success. The three factors of particular importance are: the challenges presented by the first job assignment, the actions of your first supervisor, and how well you, as an individual, fit into the culture present in the organization.

The Initial Job Assignment

The initial job assignment, and its effects on the individual, have been investigated by a number of research studies. In one study, 1000 college graduates cited their major source of dissatisfaction was lack of job challenge.[2] E. Berlew and Douglas T. Hall suggest that challenging tasks lead to the internalization of high performance standards. Those workers who are provided with unchallenging jobs have little or no opportunity to internalize high standards.[3] This information has important implications for those facilities who accept physical therapy students and employ recent graduates.

In order to develop high internalization for the profession, neither the student nor the recent graduate should be "overloaded" with routine initial patient treatment assignments. Too often, due to perceived levels of inexperience, students and recent graduates are assigned treatment tasks which provide little or no career challenge. A new graduate will quickly burn out when the organization continually "dumps" patients on them that more experienced therapists have no interest in treating.

Creating challenging jobs may also reduce the personnel turnover rate in many departments. One study indicates that physical therapists change jobs on an average of every 1.87 years.[4] A department which incurs a high personnel turnover rate will have increased costs for professional recruitment and numerous lost patient treatment opportunities.

The Importance of Your First Supervisor

Too often, the physical therapist seeking a staff position pays little regard as to who will be their immediate supervisor. In most instances, the therapist will focus solely on the facility, the rehabilitative equipment present, and the salary which is offered. A number of researchers have noted the influence the first supervisor has on a new employee's performance.[5] For the employee new to the health care organization, the supervisor represents an individual who has not only acquired a thorough understanding of the profession but also one who has the ability to direct others.

Supervisors of new employees must have insight and patience. The supervisor must be willing to tolerate a higher number of mistakes and work with guiding the individual down the appropriate career path. Employees quickly recognize whether the supervisor encourages performance and recognizes individual potential. Those employees who are repeatedly led to believe their performance is poor will often respond in a manner which fulfills the negative expectations. For these reasons you must evaluate your immediate supervisor and the ability this person has to enhance your career. Once in a position of management, remember how important it is to influence the careers of others, especially those who are new to the profession.

Organizational Culture and the Individual

An organization's culture is the shared beliefs, values, and expectations of the organization's members. The culture represents the understandings members have concerning the organization's style of work, the proper attitude of employees, and how patient care should be provided. For some health care professionals new to an organization, there will be an immediate bonding with the culture of the organization. In other situations, a lack of understanding and agreement will be evident from the very beginning. How a manager introduces the employee to the organization influences how the individual will feel about retaining membership.

Each employee should be carefully introduced to the organization and its culture. The employee should be informed about the organization's basic operations and provided with background concerning the people with whom he or she will be working. By the same token, present employees should be provided with a brief description of the new employee before their first day of work. Introducing the employee to the organization's culture helps foster a more cohesive working environment.

DEVELOPING MANAGERIAL CHARACTERISTICS

Success in the profession of physical therapy is determined, in part, by hard work, dedication, attending lectures and conferences, as well as by remaining aware of progressive theories and trends. The same is required for achieving success in health care management. The health care manager must become familar with some of the characteristics which enable the individual to stand out as a leader. The starting point for individual career planning is to understand what should set the manager apart from all other employees. The following are characteristics recommended for the physical therapist aspiring to become a top health care manager:

1) CHARACTER. The health care manager should be someone who is above reproach. Members of the department should feel as though they can confide and trust their supervisor.

2) INITIATIVE. The supervisor should be one who encourages new ideas and is willing to take risks. Providing physical therapy should not become a routine endeavor in any department. It is the supervisor's role to encourage creativity.

3) DESIRE TO SERVE. One of the important qualities of a good leader is to recognize what followers want and need. The supervisor must be willing to work to satisfy the professional and non-professional aspirations of department employees.

4) AWARENESS AND PERCEPTION. The health care supervisor is the one charged with the responsibility of analyzing what transpires in the internal and external environment of the organization. Knowing how to recognize the need to change is part of the controlling process of health care management.

5) FORESIGHT, VISION, AND INTUITION. The health care manager must be an individual who is accustomed to planning for, and anticipating future events. Through appropriate methods of planning, the manager can lessen the degree to which a decision must be made under conditions of risk.

6) OPEN-MINDEDNESS AND FLEXIBILITY. The modern health care manager cannot operate in a "intellectual vacuum" and meet with long-term success. Those health care managers who will meet with the greatest success as we approach the year 2000 will allow subordinate participation. Flexibility will be required to allow subordinates to express creativity and enhance patient treatment results.

7) PERSUASIVENESS AND EMPATHY. The days of ordering employees to comply are gone. Employees who are treated with respect will, in turn, show respect to the health care manager. The best method is to assign tasks and provide feedback on performance.

8) INTELLIGENCE. Health care is becoming increasingly more complex, requiring those who manage its delivery to act in ways which recognize the needs of the patient, the organization, and its members. Recognizing the physical therapy department as only a small part of a complex health care system forces the manager to function in an intelligent fashion.

High performance, excellent work, and staying in contact with upper management are some of the basics for a successful career in health care administration. A number of books, including *Executive Career Strategy*,[6] *What Color is Your Parachute?*,[7] *Getting Yours*,[8] *Career Strategies: Planning for*

Personal Growth,[9] *Career Success/Personal Failure,*[10] are recommended for advancing a career. Their application to the career of a physical therapist will depend on the organization and the individual's career stage.

CAREERS OVER A LIFETIME

Throughout our professional and non-professional careers, our lives will pass through a number of stages. Understanding your present life stage and where your life could be headed in the future is important to understanding why and how we manage organizations as we do. The evolution of a career has been studied by Daniel Levinson in his research on a group of men, ages 35–45.[11] His study suggests that the adult life consists of fairly predictable changes that occur every five to seven years. These changes involve a series of personal and career-related transactions which are described in the following:

Early Adult Transition (Ages 17-22)

During this stage the individual tries to become his or her own person and move away from close family ties. The individual rarely severs ties completely, since they are likely to be either emotionally or financially tied to parents. According to Levinson, those who can gradually assert their independence will be more successful in their careers than those who retain prolonged parental ties.

Entering the Adult World (Ages 22-28)

Here, individuals have completed most of their education and have selected a career. Most also make commitments towards the future. For those who are uncertain about what they would like to do, this period may be characterized by a prolonged search for a career path and direction.

Transition (Ages 28-33)

During the transition phase the individual will review progress toward previously established career and personal goals. If the individual is pleased with what has occurred, he or she will continue on the present course. If the career or personal life has not been satisfactory, the individual may desire to move, change jobs, or even seek a divorce. People going through the transition phase may look upon this period of life as one last chance to really do something they want to do.

Settling Down (Ages 33-40)

The settling-down phase is often characterized by an individual who subordinates everything else to become dedicated to career advancement and to becoming the best person possible. Friendships may be limited, or at least minimized, to allow the individual to concentrate fully on the job. The person may desire to spend increasing periods of time associating with those who can be of assistance in advancing a career.

Mid-Life Transition (Ages 40-45)

Once again the individual will assess career progress. Those who are satisfied with how their careers have transpired will generally continue on their present course. Those who are less than satisfied with their careers may experience a "mid-life crisis." Here, feelings of frustration and sadness may alter traditional behavioral patterns. Those going through a particularly difficult period may exhibit excessive drinking or possibly quit a job.

Middle Adulthood (Ages 45-50)

During this period the behaviors which were exhibited in mid-life transition have become effectively resolved. The person will desire to devote increased attention to old friendships and try to develop new ones. The individual will often desire fewer constraints at work and in their personal lives.

Transition (Ages 50-55)

This phase may be characterized by the individual's attempt to solve problems or address issues that were not satisfactorily resolved during the transition phase of 28–33 years or during the mid-life transition phase. If the individual is dissatisfied with the changes that have occurred, a moderate crisis may result.

Culmination of Middle Adulthood (Ages 55–60)

This is characterized as a relatively stable period of one's life where there is a gradual acceptance of the fact that one's career is coming to a close and retirement is impending.

Late Adult Transition (Ages 60–65)

It is during this five-year period that many people choose to retire. This can be a very happy period for the individual where they take time to reflect on a successful career and the accomplishments which have been made. Others have trouble facing the adjustments required for retirement.

Late Adulthood (Ages 65 and Older)

During this period, many people enjoy the freedom they have from work. With more free time, they often pursue such leisure activities as traveling. Many of the activities pursued are those which they were unable to do when they were younger. This period may also be a difficult time, since health problems may begin to surface.

Levinson's work provides some valuable information which helps to explain why and how our lives change. It should be noted, however, that marked changes have occurred in society since the late 1960s and early 1970s when the study was first conducted. Since that time the composition of the work force has changed dramatically. It should also be noted that the study was performed entirely on men. The increasing numbers of women entering the work force, as well as two-income families, have probably influenced the evolution of the career.

DEVELOPING A CAREER AS A HEALTH CARE PROFESSIONAL

Few of us set aside time to evaluate where we would like to be in 5, 10, or 15 years from now. For many health care professionals the typical pattern of career success has been defined as having a good job with a good salary in a position that allows the individual to exercise creativity with continued opportunities for promotion. The traditional idea is that the employee should be loyal to the organization which in turn will be loyal to the employee through increases in salary, promotions, security and benefits. It has been traditionally assumed the professional would make a commitment to the organization and would serve it well.

Increasingly, the physical therapist is looking more for job challenge than job security. In the profession of physical therapy the individual has little, if any, trouble locating a job. Professional journals provide numerous advertisements seeking therapists to occupy one of hundreds of positions available in the United States. A report recently completed by the Institute of Medicine projected demand nationally for physical therapists will rise by over 87 percent by the year 2000.[12] If this occurs, it will result in a net gain of 53,000 new jobs.

Based on the projected growth, the physical therapist is now in a position to seek and obtain more challenging job opportunities. The therapist can, as such, control much of his or her own career success. The individual may now assume full responsibility for a career direction and measure its success in terms of achievement, prestige, money, self-respect, or by various unrelated off-the-job activities.

Developing a professional career means to plan what you desire to accomplish and to manage the steps on how the career is to proceed. Planning a professional career is the very personal process of planning one's life work. To do this the individual must evaluate his or her abilities, interests, goals, as well as examining present career opportunities and predicting the future. Managing a career involves establishing a pattern of career advancement, including timetables, which allows you to reach your goals. The steps in planning a professional career should include the following:

1) A PERSONAL SELF-APPRAISAL. Here, you must evaluate what you like and dislike about yourself. This should include an evaluation of personal strong and weak points which can be used to further or hinder career development. Included in the self-appraisal should be an evaluation of the relative interest you have in assuming a management position. Each individual should also evaluate the strength of interpersonal communication and administrative skills. Conclude the personal self-appraisal by identifying what is important in your life now and how that is likely to change in the future.

2) PROFESSIONAL SELF-APPRAISAL. Performing a professional self-appraisal means to analyze your professional abilities and interests. Deciding on a professional course of action should include assessing where your patient and personal skills are their strongest. Every

physical therapist is endowed with a unique set of skills and abilities that allow a heightened interaction with some patients over others. Rehabilitation skills and interests will also vary from person to person.

3) IDENTIFY OPPORTUNITIES. When considering advancement into health care management there must be a thorough matching of individual skills and values with career opportunities. Moving into health care management can be difficult, especially if you are a recent graduate of physical therapy. Increasingly, minimum requirements for the most challenging positions require related supervisory experience and either a master's degree in health care administration, business administration, or other similar degree. A master's degree from an accredited university is likely to take two to three years, depending on course work and graduation requirements. Pursuing a master's degree in hospital administration frequently requires the completion of an internship similar to that found in the profession of physical therapy.

4) ESTABLISH GOALS. To increase the chances of succeeding in any professional endeavor, the individual must establish career goals. Those individuals who are considered leaders in health care management attain their positions of success through hard work and goal orientation. Good health care managers are in demand because they know where they have been, how they got there, and where their career should take them next. In other words, they possess drive.

Properly establishing career goals must consider the time frame under which the goal is expected to be achieved. A goal such as, "Someday, I would like to be the chief executive officer for a community hospital" is a subjective goal. The only reason this is considered a subjective goal is because it does not specify a time frame. It is not uncommon for many physical therapists to proceed through their entire career without establishing time frames for where they would like to be in the future.

To help rectify this problem, the health care professional should consider three time frame options. The first time frame is the immediate period of about one year. The second time frame should extend beyond one year to no more than five years. The second or intermediate time frame should be considered the most realistic because it can be determined with relative accuracy. Lastly, the third time frame is the period during which ten-year goals are established. Long-term goals are frequently ambiguous but are important, since they serve the purpose of keeping the health care professional pointed in the right direction. Figure 13-1 outlines each of the goal development time frames.

```
┌─────────────────────────────────────────────────────┐
│              HYPOTHETICAL CAREER GOALS                │
│                                                       │
│  IMMEDIATE (1 Year)                                   │
│  ─────────────────                                    │
│  Enroll in an accredited graduate program in Business │
│  Administration at the local university.              │
│                                                       │
│  Locate an assistant directors position.              │
│                                                       │
│                                                       │
│  INTERMEDIATE TIME FRAME (1–5 Years)                  │
│  ───────────────────────────────────                 │
│  Complete the graduate degree.                        │
│                                                       │
│  Begin facility planning for a private practice.      │
│                                                       │
│  Locate and accept a directors position.              │
│                                                       │
│  LONG TERM (5–10 Years)                               │
│  ─────────────────────                                │
│  Open a private practice sports medicine facility.    │
└─────────────────────────────────────────────────────┘
```

Figure 13-1.

Establishing criteria is the most important factor in career success. Criteria can be established with reasonable certainty for the immediate and intermediate time frames. Establishing criteria for periods beyond five years is difficult, since needs and values are likely to change. In general, the key factors to consider in the criteria development include:

1) Designating specific jobs and job titles to achieve.
2) Establishing realistic target salaries.
3) Estimating the type of jobs which must be held to reach the desired goal.
4) Estimating the number of people who should be supervised at each level of responsibility.
5) The educational requirements.
6) The requirements for a comfortable life-style.

7) The administrative responsibility desired (chief executive officer, vice-president, or department director).
8) The type and size of the health care organization.

Throughout a professional career the goals within each time frame will require periodic modification. Goals which are developed for the immediate and intermediate time frame should be reviewed on an annual basis. Avoid developing goals which place either yourself or family members under stress. The idea behind establishing goals is to create an orderly progression towards career success. No career is worth the sacrifice of family, friends, or your own personal health.

REACHING A PLATEAU

Once the health care professional has reached a number of important goals and has become established, the individual may enter a period called "career plateau." A career plateau is "the point in a career where the likelihood of additional hierarchial promotion is very low."[13] Throughout the earlier years of a career, the individual worked hard to achieve success and has now reached a point where there is decreasing opportunity to break new ground. Although not an accurate assessment, the career plateau often carries with it the negative connotation that the individual is no longer eligible for promotion or presents some inherent flaw. The negative concept comes from the widespread acceptance that a career must continue on a linear pattern in order to be successful. Figure 13-2 demonstrates the sometimes normally assumed career success pattern.

The reaching of a career plateau should not be recognized as a personal shortcoming. Reaching a plateau has been known to create problems such as a personal identity crisis. Individuals may find themselves asking such questions as "Where is my career going?" or "Who am I?" Reaching a career plateau is a normal occurrence in an organization or a profession. Individuals frequently reach a career plateau simply because there are more candidates for a position than there are positions available. It is reasonable to assume that fewer jobs will be available as one ascends the organizational hierarchy.

To overcome the problems associated with career plateau the individual must learn more about their personal values and goals. It may be that a re-examination will force the person to establish new objectives and goals or establish a new course in life. Managers who determine through

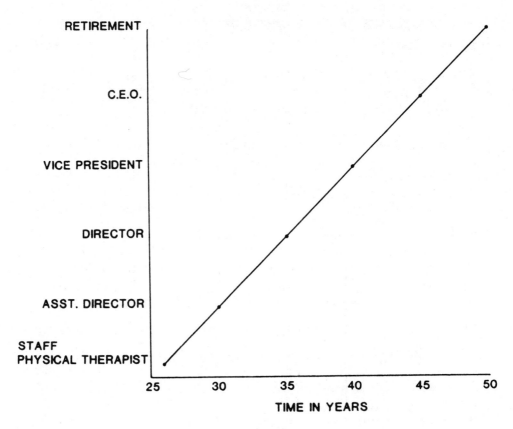

Figure 13-2.

re-examination that they are comfortable in their present positions may commit more time to the development of others. An established health care professional may, for example, show younger and less established physical therapists how to progress upward in the organization. Showing an inexperienced professional how to succeed in health care management can make significant contributions to the profession of physical therapy and to the organization.

Feelings associated with obsolesence must be dealt with on a personal level. Those health care professionals who have been in management positions for long periods may increasingly feel as though they háve become distanced from the profession. To prevent obsolesence, managers must continue to learn new skills and remain attuned to new developments in the profession of physical therapy. Staying in touch with what occurs in patient care enables the manager to more accurately forecast the future. Obsolesence can also occur due to an individual's gradual withdrawal from an area of rapid change. It can be avoided by restoring a personal commitment to remain a leader in providing innovative health care services.

PERSONAL SUCCESS IN HEALTH CARE MANAGEMENT

The decision to pursue a career in health care management can provide the professional with some of the most challenging and rewarding opportunities available in any field of endeavor. Some of the requirements for success in managerial positions include patience, drive, and the never-ending job of planning. The profession of physical therapy requires a number of additional requirements for success beyond those mentioned. They include the following:

Commitment to Hard Work

Health care professionals who work hard at their jobs will soon be recognized as valuable assets to the organization, to medical doctors, and to the profession. Being recognized as dependable and reliable is a valuable asset. Undoubtedly, your professional career will suffer setbacks, but maintaining a goal-driven professional behavior will allow you to easily overcome most obstacles encountered.

Exercise Fairness and Consistency in Management

All subordinates should know where you stand on controversial and non-controversial issues. Favoritism in any form should never be demonstrated or implied. Those managers who "play favorites" in a department will rapidly deteriorate the morale in their organization. Employees who know what is expected will be more committed to tasks than those who are unclear about how to proceed.

Remain Visible and Conversive

Those health care professionals who move up rapidly in an organization or professional association may be viewed by others as simply being in the right place at the right time. Although this may be true in some cases, it can hardly be relied upon on a continual basis. Those physical therapists who are most likely to move up in an organization or professional association are respected by members of top management and by fellow health care professionals. Most have as career goals to reach the level of success they are attaining. Managerial and non-managerial success in physical therapy requires the professional to be knowledgeable about all aspects of the profession as well as the current trends in medicine. This knowledge can only be obtained through the continual reading of professional literature and regular attendance at professional association meetings and conferences.

Control Resources

The physical therapist who can control resources has the ability to influence others. Resources come in many forms such as knowledge, ability to motivate and retain employees, or the ability to interpret and supply valuable information. The physical therapist is increasingly able to control resources through such methods as the elimination of referral for profit and the ability to evaluate and treat without physician referral. Additionally, the physical therapy supervisor who maintains a well-run department and has low staff turnover becomes a valuable asset to his or her immediate supervisor.

Willingness to Change Jobs

Health care management can present roadblocks to further professional growth and development. One of the unspoken realities for those individuals in top management positions is that they must move every two to five years in order to continue professional advancement. The necessity for repeated relocation helps to prevent the individual from becoming recognized as "organizational deadwood." A person who takes on the appearance of "organizational deadwood" is recognized by others in the organization as a marginal employee who has little or no chance for advancement. These are often individuals who have reached career plateaus and lose the motivation to perform. Carefully planned career moves can greatly enhance future advancement opportunities. The physical therapist should, however, avoid leaving the appearance of becoming a "job hopper."

Get Along with Others

Management positions involving the supervision of health care professionals can sometimes be personally frustrating. Individuals with unique skills and abilities may at times be difficult to manage. Health care managers of the future will need to become "generalists" in order to be successful. A manager who is a generalist is one who has the ability to interact with a large number of individuals with varying degrees of experience and training.

Be an Asset to Your Supervisor

Your immediate supervisor is in a position to be of assistance in planning and directing your career. Not only can the supervisor provide career suggestions, but he or she can also put you in contact with individuals outside the organization who can influence your career. Always strive to develop good relations with your immediate supervisor by providing information which can be used to enhance their own career.

Manage Conflict Effectively

One of the potentially damaging situations for a health care manager's career is a conflict situation which is allowed to continue for prolonged periods without effectively being resolved. A conflict situation which continues for long periods of time may end up being resolved by a member of senior management. When conflict situations occur in this manner, it can lower the manager's credibility. The director of physical therapy must work to reduce conflict in a department and manage it quickly and effectively when it occurs.

Accept Difficult Assignments

Moving progressively up the managerial ladder requires the demonstration of unique skills and abilities. One of the quickest ways of being recognized as an asset to the organization is to take on assignments that others are reluctant to accept. Those health care professionals with enhanced problem-solving skills increase their value to the organization and are more likely to be recognized as highly promotable by those members of senior management.

Remain Goal Oriented

Achieving success in health care management requires the same intense dedication as it does to becoming a highly skilled physical therapist. No one rises to the top of the profession and remains there without continually revising career goals and becoming a part of present and future trends. Health care managers at the top of an organization create change rather than simply becoming a part of it. Creating change requires an awareness of what is occurring in the world around you. Reading journals such as *Medical Economics, The Wall Street Journal, Business Week, Hospitals,* and the *Harvard Business Review* are just some of the sources the health care manager should become familiar with.

MANAGEMENT INFORMATION SYSTEMS

In years past, the director of physical therapy in a hospital or small private practice could keep most of the information required for running the organization in a few journals or in his or her own memory. As a result of the increasing complexity of today's health care system, the use of a simple data source is no longer recognized as being effective. Records must be kept of employee wages, days worked, sick leave accrued and taken, bonus programs, and patient treatment information. The health care organization will also desire to maintain records of costs, equipment maintenance, and productivity. To cope with increasing data and information needs, health care managers will be forced to rely on management information systems.

One of the most valuable tools for the health care manager of the future will be that of obtaining the most current and up-to-date information available. The use of management information systems is a method of providing management with timely and necessary information and reports. Managers in all organizations require information to analyze the internal and external environment, to develop strategies, make decisions, coordinate work, and evaluate the performance of employees. A management information system, sometimes referred to as an MIS, is a formalized system of individuals and machines that provide information to managers on a regular basis. The information that is provided allows the manager to plan, organize, control, and make decisions. The concept of MIS is linked to computer technology including programs and program language, terminals, and the use of storage disks.

Physical therapists in supervisory positions will increasingly need to become computer literate in order to keep pace with the changing health care environment. Computers can also be used to analyze physician-referral trends. Referrals can be analyzed from the perspective of which physicians are referring patients and what services they are requesting. This allows the director to spot potential changes in referral patterns. Practitioners can also use the data from a management information system to plan and adjust for future equipment requirements.

Physical therapists who properly utilize management information systems will make more informed decisions. Having data on hand reduces the manager's reliance on guesswork. Computer systems can be designed to provide information on:

- What decisions need to be made.
- The data required to make an informed decision.
- When decisions should be made.
- Who should be consulted prior to decision making.
- What are the current financial ratios and trends which must be considered?
- What area of the practice or department is most/least profitable?
- How services can be more efficiently and economically scheduled and delivered.

Properly using a management information system will require the physical therapy supervisor to seek additional training and education in computer operation. Becoming computer oriented is essential, since it is the manager who must manage the system. It is the health care manager's responsibility to see that the information system meets the needs of the department and that it is properly implemented.

UNDERSTANDING TYPICAL CAREER PATTERNS

Health care professionals differ in their abilities, interests, expectations, and career paths. Not all health care professionals are eager for a career that takes them up the organizational ladder. Some are content with remaining in staff positions and furthering their knowledge of patient care. A number of paths can be chosen by which to develop a career.

Understanding the varying career paths can help the supervisor direct his or her own career and be of assistance in directing subordinate career choices. Most careers can be classified into one of four categories: stable, conventional, unstable, and multiple trial patterns.[14]

The stable career pattern is one in which the individual completes a specific level of education, proceeds to enter the work force, and continues to perform basically the same type of work throughout a career. Those professionals, such as x-ray technologists, dental assistants, and secretaries, are examples of those who continue to follow the same pattern throughout much of their career. Although these professionals may change the location where they work, they continue to perform essentially the same job. Physical therapists, as a rule, follow stable career patterns. Most will have a number of jobs at various locations but will continue to provide patient care throughout their career.

The person who follows a conventional pattern of career development will hold a number of positions during the first ten years of a career. The individual will then settle into one position and follow a stable career pattern. Those physical therapists aspiring for positions in top management and as department directors will follow this pattern. This first few employment positions will be those which provide a wide variety of patient treatment opportunities. As the individual increasingly becomes more comfortable with the profession, opportunities for management will be sought. The physical therapist will hold a number of managerial positions until one is located which is satisfactory for the remainder of a career.

Those individuals who follow an unstable career pattern will initially follow the conventional path, but after a period of time revert back to a trial job and start the career process all over again. Those who experience a "mid-life crisis" may exhibit such behaviors. Still others may desire a change simply because they are tired of what they are doing. The physical therapist who displays an unstable career pattern may provide years of patient care and suddenly decide to follow another path. The individual may, for example, decide to return to school and obtain a medical degree.

A multiple-trial career pattern is unlikely to be seen in those who are highly trained in a profession. The person who follows this career pattern moves from one job to another without demonstrating much evidence of stability. Usually characterized by a low educational background, these individuals will often work a number of jobs throughout a lifetime without ever achieving an acceptable level of skill at any one job.

THE DUAL CAREER

An increasing concern for a number of health care professionals is the dual career. A dual career is characterized as a situation where both husband and wife are working. Each is pursuing a career that may or may not have existed prior to getting married. In the profession of physical therapy, where many of the working therapists are women, dual careers may be a source of family stress.

The dual-career marriage faces a number of important issues often not faced by marriages where only one spouse is employed.[15] The couple must objectively deal with the household responsibilities as well as with the problems presented with raising children.[16] Often, the husband will be expected to perform some of the traditional housekeeping duties that were once reserved only for the wife. Increasingly, the couple must deal with the stress of deciding who will stay home when the children are sick. Obviously, flexibility and a strong willingness to compromise are imperative to their careers and to the relationship.

To identify and manage some of the stresses associated with a dual career, Francience Hall and Douglas Hall have classified the four most common themes.[17] Each is based on the spouse's degree of commitment to home or career. They are:

Accommodators

The couple who assumes the role of accommodators is more closely tied to the more traditional expectations of a family. One spouse may assume the majority of the responsibility for pursuing a career while the other assumes much of the responsibility for raising the family. Neither will do so in a total sense. A physical therapist may, for example, work at developing a career on a part-time basis but be home to greet the children when they arrive from school.

Adversaries

Couples who are career oriented but also value the proper home environment may become involved in conflict situations. Neither wants to make the sacrifices they consider necessary to maintain the "proper" home environment. Each considers their career as valuable and as something which must be pursued.

Allies

Those couples who are considered as allies devote either high priority to their careers or to their home life. One will be considered as a priority over the other. If, for example, the couple decides their careers are more important, they may delay having children or, in some cases, forego the event entirely.

Acrobats

Acrobatic couples try to give equal attention to career and family. They do not encourage one another to assume a particular role. They will perform both roles themselves rather than attempting to get their spouses to take over.

Increasingly, dual-career couples are shaping the way many organizations are doing business. The U.S. Bureau of Labor Statistics reported that as many as 50 percent of all couples are dual-career couples.[18]. This percentage is expected to grow to 86 percent by the year 1990. Those areas of the country which are expected to increase the most in dual careers are the West Coast, Chicago, Denver, New York and the Washington-Baltimore area.[19]

Projections such as these have forced some organizations to offer day-care services in order to entice and retain valuable employees. Offering such services may become the wave of the future, especially for those employers of a high number of female health care professionals.

WOMEN IN HEALTH CARE MANAGEMENT

Women in health care management face the same challenges as men and sometimes many more. Although much less of a problem than in years past, women still face daily discrimination, sexual stereotyping, and increasing strains on a marriage as a result of pursuing a career. Even though many women have qualifications and abilities far exceeding their male counterparts, the factors mentioned often discourage women from entering health care management.

A number of problems face women who are attempting to enter into health care management. In some organizations, women are considered as second choices when it comes time to be considered for a managerial position. The old stereotype is that, "She may be equally qualified for the job, but where will she be when the children are ill?" Although overt discrimination against women does exist, research indicates that biases against women found in earlier studies are beginning to diminish.[20]

In response to some of the problems with discrimination against women in the work place, the Equal Employment Opportunity Commission issued guidelines in 1980 designed to curtail sexual harassment. Sexual harassment refers to any actions that are sexually directed, unwanted, and subject the worker to adverse employment conditions.[21] The guidelines indicate that unwelcome sexual advances, requests for sexual favors, or verbal or physical acts of a sexual nature that affect decisions about employment conditions, promotions, and pay raises constitutes sexual harassment.[22] Shortly after the EEOC issued the guidelines more than 300 sexual harassment charges were filed by female workers. Of the charges that were filed, 118 charges were later substantiated. The cases involved women who refused sexual advances, were fired, or were transferred to less desirable jobs. Still others had resigned due to continuing harassment.

The guidelines established by both the Equal Employment Opportunity Commission and by Affirmative Action have made the future much brighter for those women who desire to enter management. Women hold approximately 22 percent of all management jobs. Of this total, women occupy only about 5 percent of middle management jobs and about 1 percent of top management jobs. The large portion of these jobs are in areas of education, public administration, and health care. To combat these statistics, increasing numbers of women are preparing for careers in business. It has been estimated that 4 percent of the MBA's went to women in 1970 versus 40 percent in 1985.

MENTORING:
A METHOD OF DEVELOPING TALENT FOR THE FUTURE

One of the most promising methods for developing competent health care managers in the future is to implement the concept of mentoring in a physical therapy department. A mentor is a person who serves to aid the career development and upward progression of a less experienced individual. A department director who serves as a mentor is someone who possesses a thorough knowledge of the organization, the practices of management, and is willing to offer advice to the less experienced health care professional. Providing mentor relationships in a health care organization has the potential to greatly enhance the profession of physical therapy. A study of more than 1200 executives found that greater than 60 percent received guidance from a mentor who aided in their career development. Those who had mentors tended to be more highly educated, received higher earnings at younger ages, and later became mentors themselves.[23]

What can the profession gain from a mentor relationship? Those physical therapists with an interest in health care management learn not only the business aspects of physical therapy but also learn how to relate to other health care professionals from a position as supervisor. Mentoring also provides the physical therapist with a background on how to handle problems, establish a career direction, a philosophy of management, and in the development of managerial confidence.

Mentor relationships in private practice can provide the less experienced professional with exposure to the competitive aspects of small business ownership. The therapist can learn how to interview employees and make wise financial decisions. Observing a seasoned health care professional's level of maturity, philosophical attitudes and beliefs about the health care environment, ability to resist panic in crisis situations and replace it with rational-analytical reasoning all come from properly developed mentor relationships.

THE CAREER CHOICE IS UP TO YOU

Acquiring the skills to become a respected and successful health care manager is a complex activity. Developing into the best manager possible takes more than just reading this book, listening to lectures, or on-the-job experience. The physical therapist must acquire the proper mix of technical, human, conceptual, and diagnostic skills. Hopefully, some of this information will be provided through the assistance of a mentor.

A career in health care management has much to offer, including above average pay, benefits, considerable status, and prestige. Operating in a managerial setting entails the careful use of judgment and the exercise of responsibility. Lifelong learning is as much a requirement for the therapist as it is for the health care manager. The physical therapist who fails to continue to grow and develop should not consider advancement into health care management. The commitment to learn and to take advantage of all opportunities for professional interaction are just some of the foundations for a successful career in health care management.

REFERENCES

1. Alvin Toffler, The Third Wave (New York: William Morrow, 1980).
2. Marvin D. Dunnette, Richard D. Arvey, and Paul A. Banas, "Why Do They Leave?" Personnel Psychology, 34, no. 1 (May–June 1973), pp. 25–39.
3. David E. Berlew and Douglas T. Hall, "The Socialization of Managers: Effects of Expectations on Performance," Administrative Science Quarterly, 11, no. 2 (September 1966), pp. 207–223.
4. Bill Haley, "1988 Staff Physical Therapist Salary Survey," Physical Therapy Forum, vol. 8, no. 14 (April 10, 1989).
5. See, for example, Schein, "The First Job Dilemma," J. Sterling Livingston, "Pygmalion in Management," Harvard Business Review 47, no. 4 (July--August 1969), pp. 81–89, and Douglas W. Bray, Richard J. Campbell, and Donald Grant, Formative Years in Business (New York: Wiley, 1974), p. 73.
6. F. Schoonmaker, Executive Career Strategy (New York: American Management Association, 1978).
7. R. Bollos, What Color is Your Parachute? (Berkeley, CA: Ten Speed Press, 1972). See also, P. Cochran and S. Wartick, "Golden Parachutes: A Closer Look," California Management Review, 1984, 26 (4), pp. 111–120.
8. L. Pogrebin, Getting Yours: How to Make the System Work for the Working Woman (New York: McKay, 1975).
9. A. Souerwine, Career Strategies: Planning for Personal Growth (New York: AMACOM, 1978).
10. A. Korman and R. Korman, Career Success/Personal Failure (Englewood Cliffs, NJ: Prentice-Hall, 1980).
11. Daniel J. Levinson, Charlotte N. Darrow, Edward B. Klein, Maria H. Levinson, and Braxton McKee, The Seasons of a Man's Life (New York: Knopf, 1978).
12. Institute of Medicine, 1989 survey.
13. Thomas P. Ference, James A. Stoner, and E. Kirby Warren, "Managing the Career Plateau," Academy of Management Review, 2, no. 4 (October 1977), pp. 602–612.
14. Douglas T. Hall, Careers in Organizations (Pacific Palisades, CA: Goodyear, 1976), pp. 52–54.
15. David G. Rice, Dual-Career Marriage: Conflict and Treatment (New York: The Free Press, 1979).
16. C. L. Johnson and F. A. Johnson, "Attitudes Toward Parenting in Dual Career Families," American Journal of Psychiatry, 134 (1977) pp. 391–395.
17. Francine Hall and Douglas T. Hall, The Two-Career Couple (Reading MA: Addison-Wesley, 1978), pp. 22–25.

18. M. K. Levenson and R. W. Hollmann, "Personnel Support Services in Corporate Relocation Programs," Personnel Administrator, (September 1980), p. 46.

19. D. Martin, "Dual-Career Marriages are Altering American Business," Times (San Mateo, CA), February 2, 1983.

20. Hazel F. Ezell, Charles A. Odewahn, and J. Daniel Sherman, "Women Entering Management: Differences in Perceptions of Factors Influencing Integration," Group and Organizational Studies, 7, no. 2 (June 1982), pp. 243–253.

21. Gary N. Powell, "Sexual Harassment: Confronting the Issue of Definition," Business Horizons, July-August 1983, pp. 24–28.

22. U.S. Code 24 CFR 1604.11.

23. Helen J. McLane, quoted in Management World, June 1981, pp. 23–24.

GLOSSARY

ACCOMMODATING STYLE. An interpersonal style of managing conflict characterized by a lack of assertiveness concerning one's own choice of desired outcomes.

ACHIEVEMENT MOTIVE. One of the three needs as defined by David McClelland. Those individuals with strong desires to achieve spend considerable time thinking about their jobs and how they can do them better or accomplish important things.

AFFECTIVE CONFLICT. A conflict associated with emotional responses from interpersonal relations. People literally become "mad" at one another.

AFFILIATION NEEDS. The need to be social, have friends, and be accepted by others.

AGGRESSION. A reaction to frustration which involves a direct attack upon the person or barrier which is preventing attainment of the objective or goal.

APPRAISAL INTERVIEW. The final step in the employee's evaluation of performance.

APPROACH-APPROACH CONFLICT. An intrapersonal conflict situation where the person has a choice between two or more positive alternatives.

APPROACH-AVOIDANCE CONFLICT. An intrapersonal conflict situation which presents both positive and negative consequences.

AUTOCRATIC LEADERSHIP. A leadership style which is characterized by very tight repressive supervision. The manager characteristically withholds communication from subordinates and only communicates when it is necessary for the performance of the job.

AUTONOMY. The degree to which a job provides substantial freedom and independence in scheduling work and carrying out procedures.

AVOIDANCE. A method of conflict resolutions where the individual desires not to confront the problem. The avoidance style of conflict resolution may be evidenced as non-attention, physical separation and limited interaction.

AVOIDANCE-AVOIDANCE CONFLICT. An intrapersonal conflict situation where the persons must choose between two or more negative alternatives.

BALANCE SHEET. A financial statement generally developed on an annual basis that reports the financial position of an organization at a specific point in time.

BEHAVIORAL LEADERSHIP THEORY. The study of leadership that seeks to identify leadership styles that are effective in varying situations.

BOARD OF DIRECTORS. A select group membership consisting of seven to fifteen members, each possessing varying backgrounds and knowledge, who are charged legally and morally with the responsibility for the operation of a hospital or business.

BOTTOM-UP BUDGETING. A method of budgeting where department managers are responsible for developing a budget and implementing it in their own department.

BOUNDED DISCRETION. A limitation placed on decision making to consider only those decisions which fall within acceptable moral and ethical standards.

BOUNDED RATIONALITY. A decision-making situation where the available alternatives are so numerous that management cannot possibly consider them all. There is a naturally imposed limit to alternative consideration because of the complex nature of the situation and the human ability to process all of the alternatives.

BRAINSTORMING. A technique for generating solutions for a problem. A group is assembled and all members are encouraged to make suggestions. The ideas are then evaluated and a solution is chosen. The idea is to support the free flow of ideas while at the same time suspending all critical judgments made by any member of the group.

BREAK-EVEN ANALYSIS. An analytical technique for examining the various relationships between fixed costs, variable costs, and the revenues generated by the organization. The break-even point is that point where the revenue generated by providing services is equal to the cost of providing those services. It is the point to where there is not profit or loss.

BUDGET. Plans which express anticipated results in numerical terms. It is also recognized as an element of control. Budgets may be expressed in terms of dollars, personnel hours, kilowatt hours, materials or any other unit which is used to perform work.

BUDGETARY COMMITTEE. A committee generally consisting of several of the organization's department heads who help legitimize the various budget estimates so that they do not appear arbitrary or capricious.

CENTRAL TENDENCY. The process of rating an employee as only "fair" in all areas of job performance.

CHIEF EXECUTIVE OFFICER. An individual who is recognized as the highest-ranking person in authority in a hospital or similar business activity.

CLOSED SYSTEM. A systems theory concept that the organization does not interact with the external environment.

COERCIVE POWER. The manager's ability to punish the subordinate for wrong or inappropriate behavior. The influence the manager possesses is based upon fear the subordinate has that failing to comply with the wishes of the supervisor will result in punishment or other negative consequences.

COLLABORATIVE STYLE. An interpersonal style of managing conflict characterized by a desire to maximize joint outcomes.

COMMITTEE. A special-purpose group usually characterized by a designated membership, a chairperson, secretary, and a schedule of regular meetings.

COMMUNICATION. The process by which information and understanding is passed from one individual to another.

COMPROMISE STYLE. An interpersonal style of managing conflict which is characterized by each person receiving only partial satisfaction based on a give-and-take process. Middle ground is sought by splitting the differences.

CONCEPTUAL SKILL. One of the three skills needed by all health care managers. It is the ability to see the organization as a whole and recognize how an organization's various parts depend on each other and how a change in one part can affect the organization as a whole.

CONDITIONS OF CERTAINTY. The managerial decision-making situation where there is enough information to accurately predict future events.

CONDITIONS OF RISK. The managerial decision-making situation where the manager has at least a partial estimate of future events. Conditions of risk is probably the most common decision-making situation for a health care manager.

CONDITIONS OF UNCERTAINTY. The managerial decision-making situation where the manager has little or no knowledge of future events. Conditions of uncertainty is recognized as the most difficult for managerial decision making.

CONFLICT. Any situation in which there are incompatible goals or emotions within or between individuals or groups.

CONFRONTATION. A method of conflict resolution whereby problem solving is used to analyze problems and reach a solution which is satisfactory to both parties.

CONTENT THEORIES OF MOTIVATION. Theories of human motivation which examine what factors within the individual start, arouse, energize, or stop behavior.

CONTINGENCY-SITUATIONAL LEADERSHIP. A leadership theory in which the style of leadership chosen should be consistent with the tasks, individuals, and external environment facing the organization. The theory is that there is no one best way to manage every situation. Managers must find different ways for different situations.

CONTINUOUS REINFORCEMENT. A schedule of reinforcement where behavior is reinforced after each correct occurrence.

CONTROL. The managerial function of determining whether objectives and goals have been achieved. When they have not been achieved, management must take action to ensure their completion.

CONTROLLER. An individual who functions in gathering relevant data on costs and outputs that may be used in budget development.

CONVENTIONAL CAREER PATTERN. One in which the individual holds a number of positions during the first ten years of a career and then settles in to one position and follows a stable career pattern.

CUSTOMER DEPARTMENTALIZATION. A health care facility which departmentalizes by customer so as to attract and meet the needs of a particular group of customers. The organization identifies the particular group and then devises ways to attract them to the health care facility.

DEFENSE MECHANISM. A reaction to frustration where the person temporarily distorts reality to reduce tension associated with a situation. Defense mechanisms do not satisfy true underlying needs. They are considered normal reactions to situations that present uncomfortable or unfamiliar stimuli.

DEFUSION. A method of conflict resolution where a period of time is set aside to allow conflicting parties to regain perspective of the issue.

DELPHI TECHNIQUE. A group decision-making technique where the members are physically separated from each other. The manager solicits solutions to a problem through the use of a questionnaire and repeatedly re-evaluates the information provided until a satisfactory answer is found.

DEMOCRATIC LEADERSHIP. A leadership style which is characterized by a free flow of communication among group members. Matters are discussed with group members before decisions are made.

DEPARTMENTALIZATION. Departmentalization is the process of dividing the work the organization is to perform into smaller and more specialized jobs. Health care organizations may be departmentalized by function, product, territory, customer, process and equipment, or time.

DEPARTMENTALIZATION BY TIME. In hospitals, departmentalization by time is evidenced in the department of nursing. Each workday is divided into three eight-hour shifts.

DIAGONAL COMMUNICATION. The flow of messages from one individual or group to another individual or group that are not on the same lateral plane in the organization. Communication of this type cuts across functions and levels within an organization.

DIRECT ACTION ENVIRONMENT. Factors which directly influence or are influenced by the operations of the health care organization. Major suppliers, competitors, and patients are part of the direct action environment.

DIRECTIVE INTERVIEW. An interview in which the supervisor has a specially pre-pared group of questions which must be asked of each candidate. The purpose of a directive interview is to obtain enough information in order to make an informal decision about the prospective employee.

DOWNWARD COMMUNICATION. The channel of communication used specifically by management for sending information, orders, directives, policies, and memoran-dums to subordinates.

DUAL CAREER. A situation where both husband and wife are working.

DYNAMIC SYSTEM. A system in which considerable change takes place over time.

E.R.G. THEORY. A less rigid model of the theory developed by Maslow. Needs are divided into Existence, Relatedness, and Growth. In contrast to Maslow's theory, Alderfer's theory recognizes several needs may exist at one time and that basic needs may not be achieved in a hierarchial order.

EFFECTIVENESS. The ability to achieve established objectives over a period of time.

EFFICIENCY. The ability to use resources in a manner that maximizes an output for a given level of input.

EMPLOYEE ASSISTANCE PROGRAM. An employer-sponsored program for assisting workers with drug, alcohol, or marital problems.

ENTROPHY. The system concept principle whereby an organization expends more energy than it is able to replace from the outside. Unless halted, the system will eventually deteriorate to the point of no longer remaining viable.

ENVIRONMENTAL UNCERTAINTY. The degree to which the environment moves from one that is stable and simple to one which is dynamic and complex.

EQUITY THEORY OF MOTIVATION. Developed by J.S. Adams, the theory proposes a state of equity will exist in the mind of the individual when the ratio of inputs (effort) to outcomes (rewards) is equivalent to the ratio of a comparison individual(s).

ESTEEM. The fourth level of Maslow's Hierarchy of Needs. This is the individual's desire to maintain self-respect and obtain the respect of others.

ETHICS IN PATIENT REFERRALS ACT OF 1989. A bill before Congress which would impose limitations on a physician's ability to refer a patient to a facility and receive a profit for the referral.

EXPECTANCY. The individual's perception of probability that a specific result will follow a specific act. It may be assigned a value of 0 to +1.

EXPENSE BUDGET. A budget which predicts the future and projected costs for an organization or department.

EXPERIENCED MEANINGFULNESS. According to the Hackman-Oldham model of job enrichment it is the extent to which work is viewed as important, valuable, and worthwhile by the worker.

EXPERIENCED RESPONSIBILITY. According to the Hackman-Oldham model of job enrichment, it is the extent to which the person feels responsible and accountable for the work being performed.

EXPERT POWER. Power that is held by those individuals who possess some technical expertise, skill, or knowledge that gains them the respect and compliance of subordinates. The less powerful person believes the other person has more ability or knowledge.

EXTINCTION. When used in conjunction with operant conditioning, extinction is the absence of reinforcement following an unwanted behavior.

FEDERAL RESERVE BANK. The Federal Reserve helps to regulate the economy by managing the money supply in accordance with the needs of the economy as a whole.

FEEDBACK. The degree to which task completion provides the individual with information about the effectiveness of performance.

FIEDLER'S CONTINGENCY MODEL. The model postulates that a manager's effectiveness depends on two main factors: (a) the motivational system of the leader, and (b) the extent to which the situation is favorable or unfavorable to the leader.

FIRST LEVEL MANAGERS. Those individuals who are responsible for the direction of department employees and the quality of health care delivered to the patient.

FIXED-INTERVAL SCHEDULE OF REINFORCEMENT. The reinforcement of behavior after a specific period of time has elapsed since the last reinforcer was applied.

FIXED-RATIO SCHEDULE OF REINFORCEMENT. The reinforcement of behavior after a fixed number of responses have occurred.

FORCED CHOICE. A method for employee evaluation that requires the rater to check statements that are representative of employee performance. The primary purpose of the forced-choice method is to reduce the supervisor's personal bias for or against a subordinate.

FORCED DISTRIBUTION. A method for employee evaluation, often referred to as "grading on a curve." Individuals are placed in groups based on the assumption that employee performance is representative of the entire society.

FORCING STYLE. An interpersonal style of managing conflict which reflects a win/lose approach to interpersonal conflict. Characteristic elements include power and dominance.

FORMAL CHANNEL OF COMMUNICATION. A network of communication based on the structure of the organization. The formal channel extends from the chief administrator down to the lowest ranks of the organization. It includes downward, upward, and horizontal communication.

FORMAL GROUP. A group specifically created by the organization in order to provide an organized set of health care services and meet established objectives and goals.

FREQUENCY RATING SCALE. A method for employee evaluation which examines performance by quantitative choice rather than by a description of performance.

FRUSTRATION. An individual perception that the ability to satisfy a need is blocked before the need can be satisfied. The person develops tension when a barrier has been established which reduces the ability to achieve an objective or goal.

FUNCTIONAL DEPARTMENTALIZATION. The process of grouping a health care facility by function places all activities that are similar under one individual for direct supervision. This is the most common form of departmentalization in health care organizations.

GRAPEVINE. The "nickname" for the informal channel of communication.

GRAPHIC RATING SCALE. A method for employee evaluation which examines a list of traits or characteristics which are considered important for job performance.

GROUP. A collection of two or more individuals that share a common set of interests, have frequent interactions, and work together for the purpose of achieving a common objective or goal.

GROUP COHESIVENESS. The amount of attraction group members have to one another and the degree to which they are committed to moving in the same direction.

GROUP NORMS. Values and rules of conduct members have established to maintain desired group behavior.

GROUP ROLES. The expectations shared by group members regarding who is responsible for what activities and tasks and under which conditions.

GROWTH NEEDED STRENGTH. The individual's need for personal accomplishment and opportunity for learning on the job.

HALO EFFECT. The tendency of allowing one very prominent characteristic to overshadow objective and rational decision making.

HEALTH CARE MANAGEMENT. The process of coordinating human and non-human resources to accomplish the objectives and goals of the organization.

HERZBERG'S TWO-FACTOR THEORY. A content theory of motivation which identifies hygiene and motivating factors in the work environment. Hygiene factors come directly from the organization to which the individual belongs. Motivators are factors which are associated with positive feelings about the job.

HIERARCHY OF NEEDS. A content theory of motivation which focuses on the individual's attempt to satisfy their needs. Arranged in a hierarchy from lowest to highest, Maslow defined human needs as: physiological, security, affiliation, esteem, and self-actualization. As one need is satisfied, the next higher level emerges as a motivator.

HORIZONTAL CONFLICT. A form of intraorganizational conflict which occurs between departments or employees on the same organizational level.

HUMAN RELATIONS SKILL. One of the three skills needed by all health care managers. It is the ability to motivate, lead, understand, and work with other people or individuals or as groups.

INCOME STATEMENT. A financial statement generally developed on an annual basis that reports the changes that have occurred in an organization's financial position as a result of its operations over time.

IDENTIFICATION. A defense mechanism where the individual assumes the values, attitudes, opinions, or behaviors of someone they admire.

INDIRECT ACTION ENVIRONMENT. The indirect action environment consists of those factors which are less influencial on the health care organization. Although they do affect the organization, variables such as the economy and medical technology are unlikely to directly affect daily operations.

INFLUENCING. Often referred to as motivating, directing, and actuating, it is the managerial function which evokes action from personnel to accomplish the organization's objectives and goals.

INFORMAL APPRAISAL. Primarily a method of providing feedback to the subordinate. The informal appraisal follows no pattern and may cover a variety of subjects.

INFORMAL CHANNEL OF COMMUNICATION. A form of communication existing in all all organizations, commonly referred to as the "grapevine" because of its haphazard and irregular pattern of movement. It develops as a natural outgrowth of the desire for people to interact socially and communicate with one another.

INFORMAL GROUP. A group consisting of those individuals with mutual interests, attractions, desires, and needs who interact together and share a common bond.

INPUTS. In systems theory, inputs are resources such as labor, information, energy, and materials. Each of these are applied towards patient care.

INSTRUMENTAL LEADERSHIP. A leadership style characterized by a manager who ensures the department reaches objectives and goals through careful planning, organizing, coordinating, and controlling of subordinate activities.

INTERGROUP CONFLICT. A form of conflict which occurs between two groups. It may stimulate competition and lead to improved performance.

INTERMITTENT REINFORCEMENT. A method of reinforcement which may follow either an interval or ratio schedule.

INTERORGANIZATIONAL CONFLICT. Conflict which occurs between organizations. This form of conflict is generally viewed as healthy, since it is most often seen as competition.

INTERPERSONAL CONFLICT. Concerns the method and quality of interactions between two individuals.

INTERROLE CONFLICT. A form of role conflict in which the person is expected to play different roles which give rise to conflicting demands.

INTERSENDER CONFLICT. A form of role conflict where the expectations from one person or group differ with the expectations of another person or group.

INTRAGROUP CONFLICT. Concerns conflict within a group. This form of conflict will affect how the group operates, its outputs, and its social processes.

INTRAORGANIZATIONAL CONFLICT. Conflict which occurs within an organization as either vertical, horizontal, line-staff, or role conflict.

INTRAPERSONAL COGNITIVE CONFLICT. An intrapersonal conflict situation in which the person has inconsistent beliefs or thoughts that are psychologically uncomfortable.

INTRAPERSONAL CONFLICT. Conflict which occurs within the individual involving a goal or something cognitive in nature.

INTRASENDER CONFLICT. A form of role conflict in which the supervisor provides a subordinate with incompatible orders or expectations.

JOB ANALYSIS. The process of identifying what people do in their jobs and what they need in order to do the job satisfactorily. Job analysis collects information on the characteristics of a job that differentiates it from other jobs and outlines the demands to be made on the employee.

JOB DESCRIPTION. A written statement which carefully outlines the duties and requirements that are considered part of the job. The job description establishes performance standards and describes what the job accomplishes and what performance is considered satisfactory.

JOB SPECIFICATION. A brief statement which lists the knowledge, abilities, and skills needed to perform a job satisfactorily.

KNOWLEDGE OF RESULTS. The feedback the worker receives on how well or poorly he or she is performing the job.

LAISSEZ-FAIRE LEADERSHIP. A leadership style which is characterized by a minimum of supervision with the assumption that each person will be self-motivating.

LATERAL COMMUNICATION. The communication network that exists between people and departments who are on the same organizational level but who perform different functions.

LEADER-MEMBER RELATIONS. One element of Feidler's Contingency Theory of Leadership which recognizes the importance of the leader's evaluation of being accepted by the group. If the leader feels as though he or she gets along well with the group and the group respects the leader, then the leader is less likely to rely on formal authority to get the job done.

LEADER POSITION POWER. One element of Feidler's Contingency Theory of Leadership which recognizes the degree to which the leader possesses legitimate, reward, and coercive power to influence the behavior of subordinates.

LEADERSHIP. The exercise of a special influence by one member of an organization over others of the same organization for the purpose of accomplishing certain objectives and goals.

LEFT BRAIN. The side of the brain in which analytical, systematic, sequential, and verbal thought process are predominant.

LEGITIMATE POWER. Power which is based upon the individual's position in the hierarchy of the organization. Due to the individual's position in the hierarchy, subordinates believe they should comply.

LIFE CYCLE THEORY OF LEADERSHIP. A situational leadership theory which recognizes the maturity or immaturity of the followers as being important influencing factors in the manager's choice of a leadership behavior.

LINE-STAFF CONFLICT. A form of intraorganizational conflict in which staff departments become entangled in conflict with line managers.

LONG-TERM PLANS. Plans which extend beyond one year to as long as five, ten, or even twenty years in advance.

MANAGEMENT BY OBJECTIVES. A method of employee evaluation where the subordinate and supervisor jointly establish and evaluate progress toward objectives and goals. Specific end results are identified so that the level of performance can clearly be ascertained.

MANAGEMENT INFORMATION SYSTEM. A formalized system of individuals and machines that provides information to managers on a regular basis. The information serves as a basis for decision making.

MEDICAID. A joint venture between the federal government and individual states specifically designed to meet the needs of the poor.

MEDICARE PART A. A government-sponsored health care plan which covers primarily inpatient hospitalization and care delivered in long-term, skilled nursing facilities or in the patient's home.

MEDICARE PART B. A government-sponsored supplemental medical insurance covering physician services, hospital outpatient services and care provided by home health agencies.

MEDICARE PROSPECTIVE PAYMENT SYSTEM. Legislation passed by Congress in 1983 designed to fix the per-case payments for each of 468 diagnosis-related groups (DRG's). The intent of the legislation is to shift the risk from payer to provider.

MENTOR. A person who serves to aid in career development and upward progression of a less experienced individual.

MIDDLE LEVEL MANAGERS. Those individuals who direct the activities of other health care managers.

MOTIVATORS. A set of processes which sustains an individual's behavior toward the attainment of some objective or goal.

MOTIVATIONAL FORCE. The foundation of the expectancy theory. The motivational force of the individual is the sum of expectancy and valence.

MULTIPLE-TRIAL CAREER PATTERN. Characterized by individuals with low educational backgrounds who work at a number of jobs throughout a career and never gain proficiency in any one area.

NOMINAL GROUP TECHNIQUES. A group decision technique designed to stimulate creative decision making. The problem is thoroughly discussed by group members and a solution is obtained by a mathematically pooled outcome of individual votes.

NON-DIRECTIVE INTERVIEW. Sometimes referred to as a counseling interview, the non-directive interview is used when the employee wishes to discuss a specific complaint, personal problem, or as part of the exit interview.

NON-PROGRAMMED DECISIONS. Those decisions which are made for problems that are unique or have not arisen in exactly the same manner before. Rarely are there any rules, procedures, or guidelines for the manager to follow.

OPEN SYSTEM. The systems theory belief that an organization continually interacts with and influences the external environment.

OPERANT CONDITIONING. Also known as positive reinforcement and behavior modification. The theory suggests that behavior which is followed by satisfying consequences tends to be repeated, whereas behavior followed by unsatisfying consequences tends not to be repeated.

ORGANIZATIONAL CHART. A graphic representation of the organizational structure in a hospital or similar business organization.

ORGANIZATIONAL CULTURE. The shared beliefs, values, and expectations of organizational members. They represent an understanding concerning the organization's style of work, the proper attitude of employees and how patient care should be delivered.

ORGANIZING. The managerial function of assigning duties and activities to accomplish organizational objectives.

OUTPUT. The end result produced by the health care organization.

PARTICIPATIVE LEADERSHIP. A leadership style characterized by a manager who treats employees as equals and allows them to influence discussions regarding departmental policy and procedure. Information, power, and influence are all shared.

PERFORMANCE APPRAISAL. A systematic means of determining how well an individual performed a job during a specified period of time.

PERMANENT OR STANDING COMMITTEE. A committee established to meet a continuing need within a health care organization.

PERSONAL SELLING. A marketing term for a face-to-face encounter between two or more parties for the purpose of making a positive representation of an individual, organization, product, or service.

PERSON-ROLE CONFLICT. A form of role conflict where job requirements run opposite to individual values or needs.

PHYSIOLOGICAL NEEDS. The first level of Maslow's Hierarchy of Needs. Physiological needs include food, water, and sex.

PLANNING. The managerial function of deciding in advance what is to be done in the future.

PLANNING-PROGRAMMING-BUDGETING SYSTEM. A budgeting method in which each department ascertains what it is trying to accomplish and then evaluate all objectives and goals in terms of short- and long-term costs. Funding is generally projected for a period of three or more years.

POSITIVE REINFORCEMENT. Any outcome which is pleasant encourages the individual to repeat a behavior. Positive reinforcement includes such things as praise, recognition, promotions, and money.

POWER. One of the three needs as defined by David McClelland. A person with high needs for power will be interested in controlling situations and influencing others for the good of the organization.

PRE-EMPLOYMENT INTERVIEW. A directive type of interview where the supervisor questions the applicant about his or her qualifications and interest in the position.

PRIMARY OBJECTIVES. They outline the goals and end results toward which all plans and activities are to be directed.

PROACTIVE DECISIONS. Decision making in response to something the manager perceives will occur.

PROCESS THEORIES OF MOTIVATION. Theories recognizing the individual is motivated to behave based on the rewards associated with a given behavior.

PROCESS AND EQUIPMENT DEPARTMENTALIZATION. A form of departmentalization that is very similar to departmentalization by function. All activities involving certain types of equipment or specialized technical considerations are grouped together.

PRODUCT DEPARTMENTALIZATION. A health care facility which organizes by product has a complete set of health care professionals within each department. For reasons of coordination and duplication of effort, product departmentalization is not applicable in most health care settings.

PROFIT BUDGET. The sum of the revenue and expense budgets.

PROGRAMMED DECISIONS. Those decisions which are considered routine and repetitive.

PROJECTION. A defense mechanism used to protect oneself from becoming aware of undesirable characteristics.

PROMOTION FROM WITHIN. A policy established by an organization, where management positions are filled by those employees who are already members of the organization.

PUNISHMENT. When used in conjunction with operant conditioning, the application of negative consequences decreases the likelihood that an undesirable behavior will be repeated.

RANKING. A method for employee evaluation that lists from highest to lowest the performance of all employees in a department.

RATING SCALE. One of the oldest forms for evaluating employee performance. The two types of rating scales are the graphic rating scale and the frequency rating scale.

RATIONALIZATION. A defense mechanism where the individual attempts to explain away behaviors or outcomes that are undesirable or inconsistent.

REACTION FORMATION. A defense mechanism where the individual reacts by exhibiting the opposite attitudes and behaviors to a desire or area of concern.

REACTIVE DECISION. A decision and change made in response to an identified problem. In other words, the person reacts to the problem instead of anticipating it.

REFERENT POWER. The power the manager possesses based on the follower's identification with the manager as a leader.

REVENUE BUDGET. Details the future and projected income for the services provided by a specific department or organization.

REWARD POWER. The ability of a manager to provide varying benefits to others such as bonuses, promotions, or increases in pay for a job well done.

RIGHT BRAIN. The side of the brain which intuitive, visual, spatial, sensuous, and holistic thought processes are predominant.

ROLE. An organized set of observable behaviors that are attributed to a specific office or position.

ROLE AMBIGUITY. A situation in which a person lacks clear job objectives.

ROLE CONFLICT. A situation in which the individual is faced with role expectations that are incompatible with what the individual believes is inherently correct.

ROLE-OVERLOAD CONFLICT. A situation where the person is confronted with expectations from a number of sources which cannot be completed in a given period of time and still maintain quality.

SATISFICING. A managerial decision-making process whereby the manager finds a solution to the problem without first identifing all the possible alternatives.

SECONDARY OBJECTIVES. Usually developed at the department level, they are much narrower than primary objectives and serve as specific guides for performance.

SECURITY NEEDS. The second level of Maslow's Hierarchy of Needs. Security needs include safety, protection from pain, or the threat of harm.

SELF-ACTUALIZATION. The fifth level of Maslow's Hierarchy of Needs. This is the need to discover who we are and develop to our fullest potential.

SHORT-TERM PLANS. Those plans which cover a period of no longer than one year.

SKILL VARIETY. The extent to which a job requires the use of several skills or talents in the performance of an activity.

STABLE CAREER PATTERN. One in which the individual completes a specific level of education, enters the work force, and performs basically the same type of work throughout a career.

STAFFING. The managerial function concerned with the development and maintenance of the organization's human resources to fulfill the institution's plans, objectives, and goals.

STATIC SYSTEM. A system in which little or no change takes place over time.

STATUS. The position or rank an individual holds within a group or organization.

STRESS. The psychological and/or physiological response to an action, situation, or force that places special demands on the person that are potentially harmful.

SUBSTANTIVE CONFLICT. A form of intragroup conflict based on the nature of the task or "content" issues.

SUBSYSTEMS. A small part of a total system. Subsystems are usually identified as a group, department, or specialty area within a larger system.

SUPPORTIVE LEADERSHIP. A leadership style characterized by a high concern for people and a low concern for the task or activity. The leader attempts to generate goodwill by providing a friendly and pleasant working climate for employees.

SYNERGISM. Part of systems theory which recognizes the importance of viewing all parts of an organization as working together rather than acting independently.

SYSTEMATIC APPRAISAL. The formal process a health care organization uses to evaluate performance.

SYSTEMS APPROACH. An approach to the analysis of an organization that recognizes the interdependence between departments in an organization and for the need to adapt to the larger external environment.

TASK FORCE. A committee formed to deal with a specific issue, task, problem, or purpose. The group remains in existence only until its goal or objective is accomplished.

TASK IDENTITY. The extent to which the employee has the opportunity to complete a whole piece of work from beginning to end.

TASK SIGNIFICANCE. The extent to which the job has an impact on the work and lives of others in the organization.

TASK STRUCTURE. An element of Fiedler's Contingency Theory of Leadership which recognizes the extent to which a task is routine (structured) or complex (unstructured).

TECHNICAL SKILL. One of the three skills needed by all health care managers. It is the ability to perform specialized activities in a given field.

TERMINATION INTERVIEW. A directive type of interview in which the supervisor discusses the reasons why an employee is being released from the organization.

TERRITORIAL DEPARTMENTALIZATION. A health care facility which organizes by territory does so in order to reach a segment of the population which is widely dispersed and cannot be attracted by conventional methods.

THEORY X. The managerial belief that workers must be motivated by pressure applied from management.

THEORY Y. The managerial belief that people will become self-motivated to achieve organizational goals as a natural consequence of their striving for personal growth and development.

TOP-DOWN BUDGETING. A method of budgeting where top management develops the budget and then has it implemented at the department level.

TOP MANAGERS. Often referred to as chief executive officer, president, or vice president, they are responsible for the direction and management of the health care organization.

TRAIT LEADERSHIP THEORY. The study of leadership which attempted to identify a set of personal characteristics that separate effective and ineffective leaders.

TYPE A PERSONALITY. Those with Type A personality characteristics are frequently in a hurry to get things done, impatient, preoccupied with deadlines, and competitive.

TYPE B PERSONALITY. People with Type B personality characteristics have a more confident style, are less hurried, less competitive, and are less status conscious.

UNITY OF COMMAND. The management principle that a subordinate have only one superior to whom to report.

UNSTABLE CAREER PATTERN. A career pattern in which the individual begins following the conventional career pattern but then reverts back to a trial job and begins the career development process all over again.

UPWARD COMMUNICATION. The channel of communication which carries information from subordinates to superiors. The channel functions to provide feedback to management.

VALENCE. The strength of an individual's preference for an expected outcome. The individual's preference for a particular outcome may range on a scale from $+1$ to -1.

VARIABLE-INTERVAL SCHEDULE OF REINFORCEMENT. The reinforcement of behavior using an interval of time that varies around an average.

VARIABLE-RATIO SCHEDULE OF REINFORCEMENT. The reinforcement of behavior that requires a certain number of responses before the method of reinforcement is delivered. The number of correct responses will vary around an average.

VERTICLE CONFLICT. A form of intraorganizational conflict involving conflict between different levels within the organization's hierarchy.

VOLATILITY. The rate at which an organization's environment is changing.

WHOLISM. Part of the systems concept which encourages the organization to be viewed as a functioning whole and not simply as a collection of parts.

WITHDRAWAL. A reaction to frustration evidenced by a physical or mental withdrawal from a frustrating event. The person tries to get away from the area of concern.

ZERO BASE BUDGETING. A budgeting method which moves away from the traditional methods of budgeting. Under ZZB, a new budget must be developed each year from scratch, with every dollar expenditure being justified.

INDEX

311